Aphasia, my world alone

HELEN HARLAN WULF

Aphasia, my world alone

WAYNE STATE UNIVERSITY PRESS, DETROIT, 1979

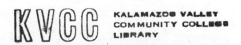

Library of Congress Cataloging in Publication Data

Wulf, Helen Harlan, 1913–
  Aphasia, my world alone.

  1. Aphasia—Biography.   2.   Wulf, Helen Harlan,
1913– I.   Title.
RC425.W84 1979   362.1'9'6855200924   [B]   79-11334
ISBN 0-8143-1646-8

For
My Balance Wheels:

HANS
My Alter Ego

and

JOSEPHINE SIMONSON
My Life-Line To Sanity

contents

foreword

Man's ability to communicate must certainly be the outstanding factor that sets him apart from the rest of the animal kingdom. Sudden and unexpected loss of communication is a terrifying, dehumanizing experience that tears away at the essence of life itself.

For decades, speech and language pathologists have sought to better understand the nature of communicative loss. The term "aphasia" is used to generally describe a condition whereby speech and language skills are partially or totally lost. Aphasia is the result of damage to or disturbance of those areas in the brain responsible for speech and language functions. A tremendous variety of specific impairments can occur to plague the individual with aphasia. Impairments of comprehension, reading disturbances, writing difficulties, and confusion with numerical processes can accompany oral language problems such as word loss, loss of sentence structure, and confusion in utilizing word forms. Often associated with aphasia is the inability to voluntarily make appropriate movements of the oral musculature (dyspraxia), or a weakness of those same muscles (dysarthria).

But to understand aphasia and its related disorders at this level alone is to miss the full nature of this terribly debilitating condition. For the effect that aphasia has on the person who must bear its consequences is a profound area of interest that is not always understood and even less seldom considered. *Aphasia, My World Alone* has been written to help open this often closed door — a door that has been opened by many others who have experienced aphasia, but never written in such a unique style, and with such profound insight.

Helen Wulf has put down on paper a depth of feeling, thought, and analysis concerning the aphasic experience that personalizes the disorder in a gripping, readable manner. She delves so deeply into her aphasia that the reader is actually drawn up into the agony and frustration that is the daily burden of the aphasic individual. The pages of this book investigate a seemingly unending stream of problems. Each problem area is unfolded and then analyzed by the author. Her ability to uncover the underlying causative factors of her difficulties sheds tremendous light on the nature of brain damage. This kind of analysis, by such a perceptive, insightful individual, is truly a rarity.

Those speech pathologists who actively work with aphasic patients will immediately recognize the value of Helen Wulf's analysis of her aphasia. Her reactions to various forms of treatment will also be beneficial, especially to those who are now allowing certain aphasics to determine which speech and language deficits are most debilitating and, consequently, which area should be emphasized in the initial stages of treatment. The author initiates a wealth of new ideas regarding rehabilitation of the aphasic that should prove most refreshing to the field of speech and language pathology.

Family and friends of the aphasic will be warmly introduced to those inner thoughts so long hidden from their ears. This book can be an excellent source of entry into the inner world of aphasia. It should be extremely useful in family counseling and will greatly aid families in the process of accepting those unfortunately permanent, remaining aphasic symptoms. As many speech pathologists have indicated, the need for "family treatment" is immediate, real, and often of critical importance. *Aphasia, My World Alone* can certainly be of value to the total process of rehabilitation.

Throughout the book, the reader will find bits and pieces of a phantom person who is responsible for allowing Helen Wulf the freedom of her analytic reasoning. This freedom and analysis must have permeated the many treatment sessions in such a way as to point the author toward her often astounding insights. Josephine Simonson is known by her students and fellow speech pathologists to be this type of remarkable and innovative clinician. Her important role in this accomplishment does not go unnoticed by the reader.

As the field of aphasia rehabilitation continues its growth and as such groups as the Academy of Aphasia persist in questioning, analyzing, and developing current and innovative diagnostic and treatment techniques, our ability to help the aphasic and his family will expand. It is felt that in its small way, this book will help make aphasia less of a world alone.

Michael I. Rolnick, Ph.D.
Director, Department of Speech Pathology
William Beaumont Hospital
Royal Oak, Michigan

preface

On February 3, 1970 I suffered a stroke. Today, three years later, I am writing this introduction to the book I wrote as soon after my experience as possible so as to make a truthful record of it. The farther away I get from the beginning of aphasia the less real it seems.

Consequently, I now read my own report in a more-or-less objective way and seem almost to be observing myself.

The reader will find much in this book to wonder about. Perhaps I can explain:

I have not written anything without having a reason for it. The reason for the rhetorical questions, for instance, is simple: in aphasia nothing is certain but uncertainty. One cannot and must not make positive statements. But the questions do need to be asked. It's hard enough trying to figure out my own aphasia. I have tried to be careful throughout the manuscript to indicate whose ideas are being expressed: that is, just mine. The only time I've said anything affecting *all* aphasics is on the final page, "every aphasic must learn the feeling of being imprisoned within himself." And that has to be true.

Subjects are repeated because they are important to me.

There are people whose identities I do not reveal; nor is it possible to clarify or elaborate on incidents when I don't know exactly what happened. I only know those same incidents had a great impact on me. They will have to be accepted as such.

Every aphasic needs to know there is something he can do, even if it's watching birds. One reason for the writing is to show that with a little imagination each aphasic can be helped to find something to occupy and stimulate his mind. I feel strongly that aphasics and every other reader should know the writing was done by me. My integrity won't let it be any other way.

Rewriting and changing hold an ever greater margin for error in accuracy. It would be easy to revamp, delete, amend, and, in the end, distort. Accuracy is one of my prime concerns, and I do not want to be guilty of tampering.

All textual editing involves making value judgments, and certain kinds of editing represent the kinds of prejudice to which an aphasic is subjected constantly. They signify another person's notion of what the aphasic meant to say, or what he ought to be thinking. Such interpretations usually come from preconceived ideas.

There is no way the writing of this book can be put in the context of a non-aphasic. When one has aphasia produced by a stroke, in all probability he will have to wrestle with aphasia the rest of his life. Recovery is deceptive. Because it has been three years since my stroke, and because I have not been wadded in a lump of depression, many people assume my recovery is complete. Actually, such recovery is on the surface. Deep down is quite another story. True, it is possible to write, to read, and to speak, though perhaps none of these abilities warrants close inspection. But internally?

Something drastic happened to me that fateful day. No longer can I cope with much of anything as I did pre-stroke so easily. Even the simplest decisions can pose difficulties. No longer can I do things fast. Noise is exceedingly bothersome. People quickly become too much. Fatigue is like an aura around me — always there. My physical and emotional selves travel in spheres where they have never been before. My mind gallops happily, but translating thinking into words or actions is a totally different proposition.

Aphasia is my current crusade. I have no personal axes to grind, but I am realistic enough to know there are many things which need badly to be told in the interests of aphasics-to-be. In relating my experiences I touch on those things. They are very much a part of what happened to me, and I would be remiss if I didn't relate all the things that had an impact on me. I may not live to see my pleas bear fruit, but given an opportunity eventually they will. More and more aphasics are found every day. May you never be among them. But those future aphasics will be helped if works like this are allowed to come to fruition.

March 15, 1973   Helen Wulf

1

The Comparative Me

Thinking is the thing I do best.
Putting thoughts on paper comes next.
Talking plods and bumps and limps in last.

Aphasia is a weird disorder made more so, regrettably, because there are those who equate speaking with intelligence. It's sad, maddening, funny, how unaware and unperceptive people can be. "Oh, so she has aphasia. What in the world is that? . . . . You mean she can't talk? . . . . Just how badly is her mind affected? . . . . . . "

My speaking sounds inebriated. I slurp and slosh and mush through too many words. But if I can't talk, I can write. And writing is nothing to the thinking I can do. It is the most wonderful fun to meander up and down the river of thought where ideas are stepping stones. A brain may be damaged, earthquaked, bashed, and yet one's mind can know the freedom of thought.

With aphasia, one is surprisingly aware that the brain, a marvelously complex mechanism, is finite, while the mind, with its grandeur, wonder, beauty and haplessly baser attributes, is infinite. To have this awareness, perhaps one may need to be submerged in aphasia, in its tortuous, unexpected, deceptive qualities which so-called normal people find too paradoxical to be believable.

For me, aphasia is an experience in revelation: an awareness of subtle nuances in human frailties and strengths; a capturing of a cosmic realization that our many layered spiritual needs may be more complex than anyone has known.

My busy life was altered forever by the stroke which slam-banged me one beautiful morning in February 1970. Interesting that I was totally unperturbed by the odd whatever-it-was that seemed to have control of me. It was an amazing sensation to find myself a spectator watching the inside — me being ping-ponged back and forth between the here-and-now and the where-ever-else. An ultimate where-ever-else victory is awing and exciting to contemplate. This was an interim skirmish.

My busy life indeed was changed. Oh, not the basics. The man whose name I wear, our children, relatives, friends have emerged from the crisis more delightful than ever. Rather, the change has been in those other ingredients that help determine a meaningful life.

Way back in the long ago the satisfying experiences of having, helping, chauffeuring and loving children had begun. Then, my energy level was high and ailments rare. When our first born became a college graduate, our second was finishing as a university freshman, and the younger duo were still in elementary school. The seasons changed at an accelerating pace until one day, almost without my knowing, yet right before my eyes, there were no little children. Numerous were the years of doings, decisions, adjustments, denouements after "desperate tragedies," and always. there were daily pleasures. There had been energy for them all.

Then, in a moment of reflection a recognizable signal was flashed, meaning that for way too long my energy output had been set on "reserve only." And how long would the reserve last? Quietly commitments were dropped one by one, until the load was lightened enough for me to manage with ease. A touch of surgery was followed by our youngest child's exodus from home for college. The lovely days of fall were spent doing even less than planned. There was the pleasure of having our home to myself, of enjoying a refreshing quaff of aloneness.

And that fall with its many renewing qualities may have

been a preparation for what was to happen midway through winter. It may easily have softened the blow, which was cushioned unbelievably by nature during the first days.

Yes, one cannot imagine how a life can be changed by a stroke without knowing something of the background of the one felled. My life had been one of having the delights of home, children, schools, related activities in number, and a growing business. At stroke time, managing our childrens' wear showroom was my chief activity, and we had just finished a January market. Market weeks, for us four major ones a year, are times when much of our selling is done. Long hours, organized confusion, sales help, a manufacturer or two, and hopefully, lots of retail store buyers, all combine to make a busy, demanding week with my niche being to keep tabs on everything.

All that is now on the periphery of my life and may always be. Right now seems too soon to be sure. If I were to tackle a market in my present "delicate" condition . . . well, it wouldn't be feasible to assume my former role. That role meant seeing that customers were graciously waited on and, if possible, calling them by their names (once names were easy, now they are slippery); knowing files backward and forward; pulling orders in a flash; quietly alerting His Nibs when things went plumb haywire; trying to keep up with orders which had to be totaled and the information recorded; and selling, if everyone else was busy and a customer needed attention. Oh woe! Selling means standing (that's kaput); showing samples (my right arm is a reluctantly coopera-tive appendage); talking about saleability, fabrics, etc. (oh dear); writing the order (slow and left-handed). Heaven help me! Thinking about it leaves me woozled by exhaustion.

No longer is managing the office my forte, so we have made other arrangements. When my rehabilitation was well under way, I was once again able to assume some responsibilities relating to the business. But, because my signatures with either hand seem to change too much too often, I cannot sign the checks to pay the bills. This has seemed odd to both Hans and me. To me, because the independence taken for granted for such a long time has been nicked. Odd to him, for in the many years of our marriage he has not paid the bills, finding them an awful chore and a grim lesson in how money evaporates. But now he signs innumerable checks without any more than frivolous comment.

Doing things at home when the spirit nudges me and at my slowpoke speed is fine. Yet there are things which cannot be done that way. My one serious disappointment has been my inability to answer a summons to jury duty. One arrived when the stroke was only two or three weeks old. Hans had me released from that without trouble, and then came another summons when the stroke was a whole year old. Misery! How could I get there and home again? How could I even sit there all day long for five days? Those many years when serving would have been easy! But no, the wheel has to wait to pick my name until it is not possible for me to come running! The second summons time I had to swear before a notary public in my own inimitable way. Next time, if it is still impossible to discharge jury duties, it may mean signing statements with my blood. Oh Goon Head and Golly Wump! It must be admitted that the stroke was an unexpected permanent roomer.

For instance, in olden days getting up was a whizbang, super speedy, slapdash carrousel of bath, dress, breakfast and off we go. Now it is a leisurely, pleasurable arising, a slow and deliberate contemplating of the day. After savoring that, there needs to be a little smackeral of something a la Pooh Bear and his honey pot, followed by a look at the newspaper. The newspaper is spread on the table and pages turned one by one as I read the important events: Paul Crume's front page column, then "Dennis the Menace" and "Peanuts." Newspapers are still a pain to peruse (lucky am I to be able to read), but I digest the Dallas *Morning News* as evidenced by the three aforementioned items. Then it is time for a luxurious soaking in a hot tub. And why not? To hurry may mean a tumble. There are lots of bruises a doubter could inspect.

Following the lobster dipping come exercises. Dull, Dull! For I cannot gallop off on a mental journey and exercise at the same time. But, even boring chores must be done and there have been very few days when I have skipped exercising.

When all those thises and thats have been accomplished I may lie down to bask in sunny thoughts. And eventually, I'm ready for whatever the day holds. Imagine! Two hours have vanished since my happy awakening and pokey bestirrings.

Socially the stroke has changed my life too. Most invitations must become a "Thank you. Better not just yet." That means not seeing friends often. But this solitude gives me time to pursue my favorite avocation: writing. And oh what luxury is a thinking day!

Now, the pressures motherhood and business dumped upon

me are at an end. If there are pressures, I impose them myself. Aphasia has demanded this of me: everything must be done step by step, one thing at a time, just one. The doing takes incredibly long, aided by nebulous energy. So I am learning the facets of slowpaced living. There are many shining ones. And it is good.

This writing is intended to share my experiences in having a stroke and aphasia, my reactions to this disorder, what episodes were distressing to me, the sorts of things that were funny, those who were and are the most important persons in my recovery. And hear this: nothing in aphasia is certain. The experiences of other aphasics may be totally different from my own.

There follow my remembrances as dictated by my memory and told in my words.

2

The First Three Days

FEBRUARY 3, 1970
The First Day

The brr-r-r-r of the alarm clock sounds somewhere in my head . . . . then it stops.

"What is today? . . . . . Oh, yes! It's Tuesday, February third, and tomorrow I'm going all the way to the Valley with Hans . . .

How odd! My right arm feels so big I can't even move it! . .

And my head! . . . .

Surely the hurting should be over by now. . .

Well, last week was awfully strenuous. When you stop to think about it, it was the first hectic week since August . . . .

How long is it going to take me to recoup my lost pep? . . .

. . . .

Hans is dressed and ready to go . . . .

Where in the world have I been? ....

How icky I feel ....

Got to get to the office and tend to things ....

Surely when I get up I'll feel better" ....

I say something to Hans — I do not remember what, nor do I know that it is completely unintelligible.

I put on a robe and go to the bathroom ....

"I can't brush my teeth ...... I can't seem to do any-thing ...... I'll take a hormone pill .... Maybe that's what I need ......Here it is in your hand ...... you know you can't take it ...... Put it back .... I can't get it back ...... Oh, just put it down" ....

I feel a wall at my back — I have no inclination to go back to bed or to sit down — I seem unable to move, mentally or physically, but without anxiety.

Terrible nausea sweeps over me ....

"Oh, don't worry — you haven't had anything to drink so probably there won't be much of anything to come up" ....

I feel myself slide quietly down the wall to the floor, my right leg going at right angles, and who knows where my left leg is.

Then Hans is beside me ....

"Why, he's worried ...... goodness, this will be over soon ...... whatever it is"

I can't say anything ....

Then ......

        I ......

                remember ......

                        nothing ....

                                until .....

                                        I

I find myself in bed.

It doesn't occur to me to wonder how I got there.

Hans is asking rather frantically, "What *is* that doctor's name?" I tell him — just jargon, as I much later learned.

         . . . .

"He's talking to the doctor ...... seems an ambulance is coming ...... now he's talking to Polly .... what is he doing that for .... after last week why bother her about this ...... he's telling her to meet us at the hospital .... well, if we are going to the hospital I'd better leave my rings at home."

So I take them off and tell Hans where to put them. He puts them some other place.

"He really is distracted."

It never dawns on me that he can't understand anything I say.

Then our son appears with a "Hi Mom."

"It surely isn't time for him to be home . . . . Oh mercy, Hans must have called him. How crazy!" . . . .

The ambulance must be here . . . . . . there are so many voices . . . . Two strange men load me onto something and carry me through the kitchen outside to the ambulance in our driveway.

"What a beautiful day! This should be a fun ride . . . . Keep your eyes closed — maybe that will make your tummy stop feeling so urpy . . . . Good night! I think they've got the siren on . . . . . of all things . . . . . . you'd think this was serious . . . . . . what a joke! . . . . Where do you think you are now? . . . . I'd guess we're just turning down Garland Road . . . . O.K., and now we're zooming into the hospital."

They cart me into the Emergency Room.

"There is Polly — the cute thing. Well, she doesn't sound upset so maybe it's a good thing Hans called her . . . . She's so darling and so sensible."

(I heard the doctor's voice but I do not remember seeing him or any nurses. I later learned that since they were unable to understand me I had attempted to write, but the only decipherable word was "headache.")

"The doctor seems to be talking on the phone . . . . We're going to Presbyterian . . . . . . into the ambulance again . . . . and here we go. This is interesting . . . . . . Thank heavens the siren isn't blaring . . . . . . That was silly . . . . . . Now where are we . . . . . . Northwest Highway . . . . at Abrams Road . . . . . . by Sterling's . . . . turning onto Central Expressway . . . . I'd go down the side road . . . . almost to the hospital . . . . on our way to the back door . . . . . we're here."

And that is all I remember until I seem to be in a hall . . . . Yes, out in the hall, where my robe and nightie and panties are replaced by a hospital gown.

"I'll have to remember to giggle with Polly about this . . . . . Do you suppose she and I are the only females who just have to have a hot bath morning and night, and wear panties to bed? . . . . . I'm uninhibited but the hall does seem a funny place to be undressed . . . . This is X-Ray . . . . there's Edison . . . . How great — a private room — what luck! . . . . Arlene is sitting beside me . . . . I guess it's night now . . . . Someone is going to do a spinal tap . . . . I've always wondered what that would be like . . . . Really no sensation — just a little prick . . . . Everyone is nice . . . . . . I must remember to tell them how wonderful they are" . . . .

Everything is a quietly come a softly go . . . . Nothing concerns me . . . . Polly is looking after Hans and Rob, or maybe it's Arlene and Edison . . . . Life is in the here one minute — the far away the next . . . . . . How good . . . . How very good . . . . to sleep . . . .

So Near . . . . So Far
The Second Day

The first three days of this episode I seem to have been taken care of by disembodied personnel.

Although I am told that many tests were made the first two days I remember almost nothing of them, nor do I recall any doctors or nurses, and I rarely remember hearing them, but what I was thinking — when my mind was percolating — is strikingly clear.

My living in this world is very fleeting — a come and go sort of thing. I am in a care-free limbo — nothing touches my consciousness enough to linger very long.

Late afternoon or early evening of the second day we learn that X-rays are to be made right away. They tell me an anaesthetic will be given which sounds a touch peculiar, but far be it for me to be disturbed about it.

Supper has just been brought to me and there seems to be relief that I haven't eaten any. And there is some conversation about my right hand which has decided not to function any longer — or was that conversation that noon?

A stretcher comes. I am put onto it and amiably off we go when . . . .

suddenly . . . .

there is a blaze of light
bright and clear . . . . . .

It's all around me . . . .

beautiful . . . .

lovely . . . .

My mind comes alive . . . .

"Surely the nurse must see it. No, I don't think
so — there'd be some sign . . . . . . It's my own private mystery . . . .
The light's all around me . . . .

and inside of me too . .

Wonder of wonders! . . . .

It can mean only one thing! . . . . .

I can go through the invisible curtain to the next plane!
This is the right time! . . . . .
I know it is! . . . .
Can anything be more exciting than this! . . . . .
No longer an ailing body to be deferred to . . . .
What absolute heaven! . . . . .
I better hurry . . . . . so many things to do . . . . so much to
learn.

The thrill of learning unhampered by this human self
. . . . What fun to plant ideas in receptive minds . . . . or
more fun even in those that aren't quite ready . . . .

And then there's
My Dear . . . . . .
Has it really been that long? . . . . . .
What a blessing . . . . .

no regrets for any of that loving
time . . . .

any of those thirty-four
years . . . .

He'll be all right . . . .

that dear realist . . . .

Will he remember the ones we talked about for another
wife? . . . .
Well . . . . I can get him to think about it . . . .
Those precious children . . . . the delights of this life
. . . . wonderfully different . . . . they've been such fun
. . . . they'll be all right too . . . . I can get to
them, and for Pete's sake, Dolls, this is as easy a time as any to go . . . . .

Or, can it be that it's easier for me? . . . . Is that why
I'm detached from you and your father? . . . . Or does being so

close to leaving this plane make that possible?" . . . .

        My thoughts are interrupted when I am told to crawl onto a table.

        "Well, honestly, how do they expect me to be very efficient when part of me isn't working at all . . . . You'd think they could see the wonder that is happening to me . . . .

        an electric excitement that's sparkling
        all around me
            and through me . . . .
Maybe dying isn't like this to everyone . . . . . .
        of course it isn't . . . . . .
           it's personal and private . . . . . .
        an exquisite iridescent bubble
           of time . . . .
Be still . . . . . .
        be very still . . . . . .
and feel
        the vibrant anticipation . . . . . .
        the ineluctable eagerness
filling every
        nook
           and
                      secret place
of your mind . . . .
So close am I . . . .
        so close . . . .
There's the rest of me — just a little ahead —
        Laughing and beckoning to me . . . .
The composite of all the ones I have been . . . .
And when this me is added —
        to be a glorious free mind —
I'll have time to figure out where I am in the eons of development . . . .
        so much to learn . . . . . .
        so very much . . . . . .
        I'm ready . . . .
How can people really wonder what
        being born
           and
               dying

is all about?

Gas! . . . .

        Ugh! . . . .

                How I hate it!

Exhilaration lifts me

                up —

                        up —

                              free . . . .

Marvel inexpressible . . . .

        laughing and beckoning . . . .

        floating through . . . .

           radiance . . . .

Nothingness . . . .

. . . .

        Irreparably . . . .

        consciousness returns . . . .

        air blowing in my face . . . .

           tummy rolling . . . .

Silently I scream —

        "No! This cannot be! It just can't!"

        It is.

"How do I drag

        HOPE

        from a pit

           so deep . . . .

it has

        no beginning . . . . .

        no end . . . .

        HOW?"

Close by I hear a nurse say, "Come on, Mr. So-And-So. Come on — wake up. Your surgery is all over and you're in the Recovery Room."

Poor guy! Silently I say, "Go on and sleep, Mr. So-And-So, 'til you're darned good and ready to wake up. You'll probably hurt anyway. What's the good of knowing that until you absolutely have to."

"No — No — right back where I started with this old urpy, hurting carcass . . . . I'm sick of it . . . . I'm tired of never really feeling peppy . . . . There's so much to be done . . . . Why . . . . oh why . . . . am I still here . . . . There just must be some reason . . . .

You're supposed to be glad . . . . . grateful . . . . . humble . . .
blah, blah, blah! Well, I'm not . . . . I hate it!" . . . .

Disappointment engulfed me — completely —

real . . . . . .

abrasive . . . . .

despairing . . . . . .

palpable . . . .

"How can disappointment be so heavy? . . . .

Push it off . . . . It won't do you any good . . . . . .

I have to go to the bathroom . . . . . . Can anything be more
earthy . . . . . Nobody has to wet oftener than I." . . . .

Back in my room again —
"Why can't I tell them what I have to do . . . . . . Could I make it to the
bathroom . . . .

. . . . I doubt if I can even get out of bed . . . . That sweet
nurse — she knows — thank heavens . . . . . . How do I tell Hans and
Rob to go home . . . . . . I sound so cross.

Now that I'm perched on this danged bedpan I can't go I
can't tell the nurse that I had — oh whatever I had, and I'm not going to
let anybody use a something or other . . . . If I have to live I'm not
going to have a — oh well, what am I not going to have I
can't think another thought.

She's turned on the water . . . . ooh at last . . . . what a
relief." . . . .

Extreme fatigue mercifully overtook every single bit of me and I
remember nothing more of that night.

Swinging From Despair to Resolve
The Third Day

"I've been gone . . . . . Where do I go so much? . . . . I've got
to think about what's happened to me . . . . I haven't heard anybody say . . . . I guess I've had a stroke . . . . It must be something like that . . . . This speech trouble . . . . what is it
called . . . . I just can't remember . . . . I understand what
they're saying to me . . . . maybe it isn't too bad . . . .

It's the going and coming that bothers me . . . . What if I
stop coming and I'm a vegetable? . . . .

Will Hans know I really meant it when I told him never to let
people feed me just to keep me alive . . . . that's a horrible thing

to do ....

I believed Mother and I made the decision ....

But for Hans to have to buck a hospital ...... They seem to have a peculiar attitude about death ...... Heavens, so do people ...... It will depend on the Doctor...........

Who do you suppose he is .... I don't seem to have seen him .... That's absurd .... odd what you think you can tell by their eyes .... if they're sad you know how much they've seen .... how much they've taken on themselves .... they're awfully special ...... Some have eyes that always twinkle and that's a good sign .... Some are as cold as fish .... Yuck .... What in the world made me think of all this anyway?"

....

"Here's Cliff (our minister). He's great and funny and understanding .... What is he doing? ...... Oh no, he can't be .... and I can't talk .... Oh no, I can't be crying, and I can't stop, and Hans is telling me that everything's going to be all right, whatever that means ...... Well, anyway the praying stopped ...... Please don't pray over me ever again ...... I don't think you even believe what you said .... But what did you say? .... How can everyone be hoping I'll live any old way .... That's dumb and stupid and cruel .... Why waste any prayers on me ...... Why not pray for the boys in Vietnam and young mothers and young fathers and young people .... but why me? .... I've lived long enough anyway, and I can't stand for the end of my life to be a burden." ....

And gratefully I floated off again.

....

"I wonder how many questions I've asked Hans .... his answers are strange .... (Later I learned that I had not tried to talk all afternoon. He had tried to answer the questioning in my eyes.)

Hans seems awfully relieved .... wonder where he's been .... he says we're being turned over to a − − − well, another doctor .... the one we were sent to is a surgeon and I don't need surgery .... oh goodness, what is this all about .... it seems to please Hansi so I guess it's fine ....
we'll get to see the new doctor sometime today."

....

The doctor came that evening . . . . the first person, other than those I knew, whom I remember. He explained what had happened and I understood . . . . . . I did not remember what he had told me although I was aware that he had given me an explanation.

He had me say "yes" and "no," which I'm assuming I did, and then he asked me to try "Methodist Episcopal," which I must have massacred. He told me when the speech therapist would be coming, and her name, and that the next day he and a nurse would come to see me about rehabilitation. He said he would start me inhaling something to jog up my brain cells.

He wanted to know if I could get along without company and I somehow gave him an affirmative answer. I wanted to tell him that I had been brought up to think that hospitals were to get well in, and not to entertain company.

How much more was discussed I have no idea. When he left and Hans left for the night I could think quietly alone . . . .

"So this is the verdict . . . . I'm not going to be a vegetable . . . . and you'd better put your disappointment plum away . . . . . . Dying is a thrill you'll have some day . . . . . . but right now you'd better get well as fast as you can . . . .

What did he mean about the extra room in my head? He couldn't possibly have said that . . . . I need a speech therapist in the worst way . . . . I'm so fuzzy . . . . I'll be so glad when she comes . . . . Maybe when I start thinking clearly I can figure out what I should be doing . . . . Your mind may be the only thing that functions and you'd better use it well . . . . that'll keep you from being a parasite . . . .

I hope they'll let me sleep until she comes . . . . How can I be so tired? . . . . What is her name? . . . . What is his? . . . . I don't think I can wait for her to come." . . . .
. . . .

3

An Unfamiliar Life Begins

The first three days! Three days during which it was decided I should give ye olde earth planet another vigorous twirl! With that decision made, I slid into recovery and rehabilitation. This account is not a recital indicating the absolute verity of the happenings. It reveals them as dictated by memory.

For me, this groping time was attuned to learning and adapting, and my approach to unfamiliar facets reflects my experiences, my feelings and my earnest thought. To this end are discussed:

The mesmerizing pattern of aphasia or is there one?

A rampant disorder of aphasics: misunderstandings.

Death viewed as a transition.

Is there a pattern?

Strokes can cause many kinds of accidents inside one's head

but, like the proverbial bull in a china shop, probably no two victims suffer identical damage. Therefore, those working with aphasics cannot pick out a pattern, a textbook pattern as it were, and hope to jam the patient into it despite any resistance on the part of the aphasic. For this very reason, in my considered judgment, aphasia appals many professionals, a feeling easily conveyed to the patient.

There is the old jingly rhyme telling that little girls are made of sugar and spice and everything nice, while little boys arrive replete with rats and snails and puppy dog tails. This is no sillier than for an aphasic's caretakers to decide how he should behave and be nonplussed when he does not.

For example, take me, an aphasic. Am I typical? I am optimistic. I giggle at outlandish things. I hate housework. I love babies. I delight in watching the backyard flora and fauna and don't whoop over digging in a garden. I find enthusiastic, perking minds a tremendous stimulant and rippling water or a fire glowing on the hearth a lovely soporific. I think food is often a bore but consider books essential to good nourishment. I find my children captivating. I am still crazy about the one with whom I joined forces those many years ago. No, I am not typical and neither is anyone else.

Let us assume, for the sake of argument, that a stroke caused identical damage in ten cases. Those ten people would be so different in abilities, talents, age, responsibilities, reactions, family make-up, qualities innumerable that the impact of a stroke could not possibly be the same for any of them.

Aphasia became for me an interlude when faculties, not consciously thought of for years, were honed to meet my needs: my ears to note inflections and the quality of voices, exasperated, friendly, patronizing, interested, anxious, loving; my eyes to watch expressions on the faces of those around me, compassionate, disinterested, annoyed; eyes for seeing covert glances of one to another; eyes to look for gestures which can be wonderfully expressive; eyes to search other eyes; eyes to see smiles with their sunshine and healing. These were moments when my thinking about myself and My Dear had to be revamped, times when my special genie was summoned to sprinkle blessings on my inner composure.

Misunderstandings

A hospital experience becomes a medley of all sorts of

incidents, and even the not-so-good ones can be lessons in humor and tolerance. Let us begin with misunderstandings which are universally distressing, since communication can be faulty normally, but for aphasics they pose a perpetual disorder which may assume monumental proportions.

Two types of misunderstandings descended upon me: one involved words said *to* me and the other concerned words said *by* me. The first category consists of three incidents involving words my bing-banged brain treated strangely. With an aphasic, it is hard to see how this kind of misinterpretation can have been done deliberately; and to be told "you failed to listen" hardly insures happy harmony.

This presents a situation in which the patient has to have his sense of humor poised and ready to come to his rescue. It is one where he finds himself in a foggy area of bewilderment with layers of murky mixed-up directions given, statements made, questioning looks darted, an area where the only beacons of clarity are smiles and hopeful, loving voices.

The three misunderstandings reported here, involving words said *to* me, were funny, dismaying and disconcerting. The funny one was on the night the doctor gave us his wonderful explanation of what had happened to me. It was really impressive: succinct, simple and thorough. Now why, by all that is good and holy, should I be unable to recall any of that excellent explanation, and remember only something he could not possibly have said: that there was an "extra room in my head?"

Little did he suspect that he had given me the most charming retreat anyone could have. By the time my stay in the hospital was over, that room was well lived in. It was furnished with one of my special secret delights, a unique oriental rug, had books everywhere and a fire crackling merrily on the hearth. It was a tower room with encircling windows looking on nature's most serene scenes: snowcapped mountains and meandering streams, sundappled woods and restful meadows, and flowers splashing their lovely colors everywhere. Oh, how peaceful it was! My controllers, if that's a proper cognomen, might have called this saving retreat, had they known about it, an escape from reality. But, to me, my imaginative escape hatch was a sure way to retain equanimity.

The dismaying misinterpretation of words with its resultant sad misunderstanding involved a pastoral prayer given by a man of whom I am very fond, for whom I have the greatest respect. This minister has been known to me for a long enough time and well enough for me to be cognizant of the kinds of prayers he delivers. He could not possibly have said the words I thought he said. But I remember no words. Only a sinking feeling of stark despair.

Unfortunately for us both, that day he happened to come at a time when ideas were whirling in my mind on how Hans could extricate us from an apparent mess. In essence, the minister's words seemed to cut off every exit to release. But how or why his words did that I know not. I do know that there were many disturbing thoughts charging around in my muddled head. There were no words, only an inexplicably disheartening sensation.

The importance of this incident is that those caring for an aphasic must be aware of and alerted to the fact that parts of the patient's communication system may be playing downright diabolical tricks on him. If one understands that an aphasic sometimes uses words he didn't intend to use and may not even realize were said, is it difficult to know he may also interpret oddly words that are said to him?

The third misunderstanding was disconcerting, a problem in perplexing linguistics. I thought we were told that I had no brain damage, not any, none whatsoever. If my brain wasn't damaged what was causing my right leg to respond only reluctantly, my right arm to be a lunky lump, my speech a weird nothing and my thinking so fuzzy? Was the doctor telling me that my imagination had produced these disabilities? If that were true why should physical and speech therapy be on the docket? Why not a psychiatrist? Why this stuff I'm to breathe? Isn't it supposed to pump a bit of life into some tiny capillaries? Didn't the doctor mean my mind wasn't damaged or was the word *mind* used? No, the word was *brain*. People often use those words interchangeably, but wouldn't he have used the proper word?

After puzzling about this so long that it was glued to memory, I decided that the stroke was real and that this was much ado about a word. Why should that have bothered me? Maybe it was proof that if one has aphasia his mind is intact. The culprit is his brain. Translating thoughts into acceptable words becomes, for some, an unscaleable peak. I early learned there is a mountainous difference between somehow asking for a glass of water, and wanting someone to sit down for a pleasant discussion about the esoteric meanings of the mind and the brain.

These examples of faulty communication should show how bewildering aphasia can be. The insulation nature provides, to protect the patient from the buffeting he receives because of the errors his brain makes in decoding, lasts only a little while. After that he must have access to his own private hideaway where he can go to be immersed in the healing waters reserved for a bruised and tired spirit. When those attendant upon the aphasic watch as shades are drawn over his eyes, please let him go. It may have nothing to do with the people around him except that they are *there*. In adjusting to aphasia the patient also has to adjust to incredible frustration and he needs, oh, how he needs, the balm found only in the quiet of the infinite.

Misunderstanding also comes from others' erroneous interpretation of the aphasic's behavior. Since aphasia has moved in with me, my thoughts often stray to the plight of those little children who seem constantly bewildered by the actions of adults. They do not know what they have done that was wrong, or what is expected of them. They, too, are wandering in a morass of perplexity. They are quite defenseless.

But an aphasic adult should not have to be so defenseless. He has a background of experience, education, work, responsibilties and character. Yet misunderstandings come to him too. Some of them he is aware of even though he cannot find the words with which to smooth them out. Some of them he senses are there, but he cannot remember what caused them. Some may be so deeply hidden they will never surface, or they may be found after a lot of ferreting. Maybe the misunderstanding is the aphasic's doing, and it is often lots easier to blame someone or something else than to assume the blame himself.

For the length of my hospital stay I sensed a misunderstanding with two staff members about what I knew not. It was felt through attitudes, looks, words I thought were spoken, facial expressions, gestures, all these indicated disharmony to me. Sometimes I seemed close to the solution only to have a door slammed noisily in my mind. Finally, eight months post-stroke, the answer popped up one day when it was least expected. It came with such clarity as to force me to relive those devastating moments. It was my fault.

Once upon a day, when the stroke was very new, I was curled up in a ball, the fetal position, a term which often refers to a dumb bunny fizzle poop who won't face anything. When my feet are like ice I'm cold all over, which is the way it was. In addition, there was an ice bag around my neck. Oh, how good it would have felt to soak in a hot tub! Physically, I was miserable: the pervading cold, a headache, an uneasy tummy. To make me feel better, my ailing carcass was bid adieu, and I slipped easily into the comforting beauty of an experience that had been mine briefly two nights before. How lovely to float in the radiant softness of light, buoyed by the enchantment glimpsed, knowing that dying is the ephemeral transition from one plane to another. These were tantalizing peeks at such consummate beauty and strength that they will surely sustain me all the rest of this life.

At this moment, when my various selves were in different realities at once, two of the hospital personnel came into my room. "Well," I thought, "wouldn't it be nice to tell somebody about a marvelous feeling. Why not these two?" Forgotten was the painful fact that I couldn't talk properly. With considerable internal enthusiasm I plunged into a description of an experience without peer. Too late the truth flooded through me! My speech was almost unintelligible! I could not communicate! But I had used one word they had understood. How did I know what the word was? Because it was obviously unacceptable to them both. The word was *die*. How did I know it was verboten? For one thing, my very genes seemed to tell me that one didn't use that word in a hospital. God forbid! And then, it is amazing the numbers of instantaneous reactions one has and receives from others. Two immediate reactions were conveyed to me: one of utter ennui; the other of fear.

Only a moment! But what a disaster! The fury I felt at myself, and no way to explain it, was great enough to cause brief tears. My fate thereby was sealed. My automatic defenses decided that I should never again mention to anyone in the hospital what was to me an experience of melding into a zenith of comprehension and wonder.

The moment when I was eager to share an experience became very nearly the same moment when the realization of my inability to communicate normally literally bombed me. It must have been then that my self-respect was delivered a tottering blow. These two people just happened to be there. It is true that their reactions seemed real to me, but it is hard to measure how much of the distressing impact of the incident was due to the awing discovery which gave my ego such a jarring punch.

Surely it is in the best interests of any aphasic to surround him with loving and intelligent support and hold in abeyance any on-the-spot interpretations of his behavior or words. Neither can be taken at face value, and there must be other than brief statistics on which to elicit a profile of the patient as a person. An aphasic should never have to feel ashamed of, and therefore unable to mention, his aphasia. How many people around him feel this way?

Do you have any idea what it feels like to realize you have been bereft of the ability to communicate as you have always done? Where do I find the right words? No clinical, objective, dissective dissertation will do. Aphasia can be a devastating trauma striking with unwarranted violence at an essence of the humanness of man: his self-esteem. How well the patient is able to adjust depends, at least in part, on how well he knows himself.

Explorations

Aphasia delivers a crippling blow to that part which our culture proclaims to make man a thinking, bright human being: the communicative arts. Whether the damage is slight, moderate, or total, no matter what his difficulties may be as he tries to express himself verbally, his mind is whizzing around at a lively pace. Make no mistake about that. Perhaps it is easier if one's mind is trained, if one is interested in constant learning and is adaptable to changing conditions. There are those who disagree with this thesis, but I am very glad to have been trained in ways that have allowed me to travel, mentally, in many exciting directions, aphasia notwithstanding.

Can one hope to emerge from this harrowing encounter without any number of bruises to his self-respect? Because of these bruises an aphasic is often referred to as self-centered. And that is purported to be condemnatory, for we live in a society dedicated to physical perfection which tends to reject those not fitting the pattern. Methinks it behooves those of us who do not fit to demonstrate the wonders that can be found in unexplored areas.

There is, for example, an awing beauty in death, in coming close to it, and that may be a startling fact to many, since people are reluctant even to think about death much less discuss it. There are those unable to imagine that anyone can feel anything but distress about dying, and when the thought is expressed that dying is an exciting moment of leaving one sort of existence for another, many view the thinker as a prevaricator or too far out to be sane. How many of you have had the experience of being close to death, of feeling that marvelous psychic pull toward a consciousness not readily acknowledged on this side of that invisible curtain? Who is to say it was unreal, that it didn't happen, that it was due to drugs the patient may have had?

Who is to contest my idea of death or yours? We are not yet equipped, apparently, to conduct courses on "Death: Hearken to Its Promises," although there are a few brave souls who felt it worth discussing from the patient's point of view. We ought not to be embarrassed by a concept which may someday be considered our birthright rather than our inevitable complete finale, nor should we feel that our culture has consigned us to the belief that dying is a subject people don't talk about seriously if they have any sense. It makes too many of us too uncomfortable. After all, it is in a totally personal realm. And maybe that's what makes it so exciting! We can dip our toes in the waves of ideas, or we can plunge in and find ourselves miraculously buoyed by ideas most meaningful to us.

So it was that, transported by the beauty of a transition still to come, I began to learn the A B C's of an unfamiliar life. I began, too, to understand how many people are involved in helping a stroke and aphasic patient adjust to an entirely different way of living. With able assistance, how I mended and progressed seemed pretty much up to me. And on those terms recovery melted into rehabilitation.

4

Rehabilitation :   Fun, Follies, Foibles

Briefly, a rehabilitation team should revolve around the patient who is the pivot, the hub of his team's activities. The function, hopefully, is for the team to be the propellant which gives the aphasic enough momentum to find a happy, meaningful life once more.

If you were an aphasic how would you want the rehabilitation team to make you feel?

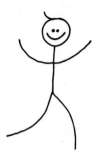

Happy Hooligan
yea Team!

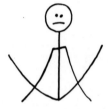

Listen,
Loony Lumps,
I'm not a thing
I'm a human me!

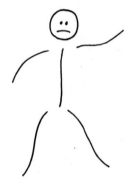

Stop pushing
and pulling,
I'm all apart
Is that helping?

I've had it!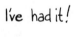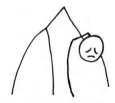

The arrangement below illustrates the composition of my rehabilitation team. There will follow a discussion of these disciplines strictly from my point of view. I bring no professional expertise to the evaluations but I do bring my own experiences. Those experiences should result in a common sense approach to a subject of primary import to a stroke patient: rehabilitation.

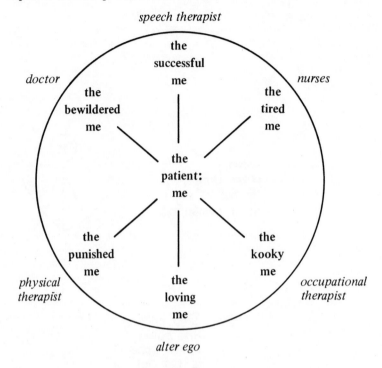

The Doctor

The doctor is of utmost importance, it seems to me, during those days when the patient is floating in a carefree nimbus. When the asphasic slides into the recovery period the doctor probably sees him daily, prescribes medication and treatments, but may not have much more than brief contact with him.

Assuming the doctor may have been the patient's physician for a considerable length of time, his role in the patient's rehabilitation may be a vital one psychologically since he is apt to know what can be expected from him. A neurologist to whom the patient has been referred, but who has never seen him prior to aphasia, will do what needs to be done, although his rapport with the patient may be tenuous, depending on any number of factors.

Whatever his relation to the patient, the doctor should know exactly how he is progressing and why. This is where the team element of rehabilitation is so important. This is where it is necessary that someone be available to determine the doings and observations of each discipline, condensing the data into a concise profile in order for each member of the team to have an overall picture of the aphasic.

Nurses

What a boon it is to any aphasic to be cared for in a stroke unit by nurses whose attention is riveted to stroke patients only. There were some absolutely superlative ones on duty during my stay. Their spontaneous smiles, their deft touches, their interested concern make the memory of that vital month a happy one.

There was one whose obvious intelligence was wreathed in a dimpled smile that put a glow into every day, and one whose bubbling enthusiasm for her work made having her near a distinct pleasure. There was one with the most unusual knack for making me feel fine. She did not have as many outward smiles as some, but she accomplished her missions with finesse and upon leaving was apt to say: "You've made me feel better now that we've talked about it." (The "it" being whatever she had told me about, and my guess is that I attempted not one word.)

There was a young concerned nurse whose potential shone clearly through her serious mien. She was marvelous for that wing because she never hurried a patient (at least not this one) and her rapport was excellent. And memory says not to forget the cutie who was as efficient as anyone needs to be, who was fast and busy, busy leaving me comfortable, amused and breathless.

On the day of my home-going a nurse came by to wish me luck. She told me she was not a regular on that floor but had been there when I was admitted. Why had she come to tell me au revoir? She gave me such a compassionate, penetrating, knowing look, a poignant, sad, sweet smile. Would I ever know what had prompted her thoughtful visit?

There was a competent nurse who never said one word more than she had to, but whose duty it was to come in each morning around the crowing hour of 4, turn on lights, do what she came to do, and swoosh out leaving the door open. (A patient's door is to be left open. Mine was to be shut a la cantankerous, private me.) It was undoubtedly a necessary routine, but often there was no return to dreamland until just before being awakened for the day's festivities.

My room must have been close to the nurses' clubhouse, and that is assumed to be an educated guess since the happenings usually occurred when night was well under way and most company had long departed. Cigarette smoke floated into my room on billowing, nauseating waves. Sadly, smoking still affects me adversely which may not be too unusual for I have never smoked. Amend that to chewing pipe tobacco at ten and smoking one cigarette when a gangling fifteen. So right now when I'm fussing at an incomparable nursing staff, maybe this is the best time to confess to things which might have caused considerable consternation if the nurses had been aware of them.

For instance, how about using cranberry juice as a tonic for azaleas? Once upon a hospital time my choice of a nightcap was cranberry juice. Only how could I ever find that word? Suddenly, the light flipped on in my head and the word *turkey* exploded, so naturally the nurse knew what was being requested. A huge glass of the appropriate red stuff was sent to me every day. It wasn't carried on the cart that was brought around each night, so it was presumed that it was sent because it had been ordered once after much struggling for the word.

After several days of tasty cranberry juice I tried to indicate that a change was in order, but over my protestations this big glass came every day. It grew larger daily and my affinity for it grew smaller until one day desperation suggested it was bound to be a good thirst-quencher for azaleas. They thrived on it, my conscience refused to hurt, methinks no one was the wiser, and the tonic continued to come up to my departure for home.

One afternoon in the hospital as I was ruminating from the bed on the scene from the window, all of a sudden the scene changed to the floor looking under the bed. How could a nutty "ageable" female have fallen out of bed? Luckily for me the door was on the far side of the bed. It was open and the only real jolt I got was when a tall, young woman walked down the hall and peered in. She had such a distracted look it seemed impossible that she had seen me or maybe she thought that was a comfortable place to sit since it was carpeted.

What to do? How in the world does one manipulate a carcass that refuses to cooperate? Well, they had been telling me to do things by myself and, so help me, I was determined to get up without anyone knowing of my tumble, and I did it! How, I've no idea. It was bound to have been an act of sheer nerve and no sense, judging by the length of time it took for my panting to simmer down to plain vanilla breathing. Even now getting down to or up from the floor is no mean feat. The incident was very funny when enjoyed alone, but I'm not sure, had this misadventure been discovered, that my pride was sufficiently hearty at that point for me to have been able to contend gracefully with a mishap so idiotic. The trauma of aphasia has many curious facets.

My experience with the floor personnel warrants the assertion that nurses are of a special breed to be good with aphasics. They need to be equipped with sensitive radar tuned to perception, and to have a sunny smile which provides the patient with infinitely more security than an unsure touch or a misspoken word. Competent, confident nurses become a sturdy bridge linking seriously ill days to recovery time to rehabilitation. They are vital to the patient's attitude toward an illness affecting one as totally as aphasia.

Physical Therapy

Because I had a few right side residuals, physical therapy was extremely important if that hand and arm were to be better than nothing. The leg was never too bad, although it still is apt to drag or stumble if not told what to do. Exercises have been done regularly every day, but they are so dad-blamed boring. They wouldn't be if aphasia permitted me to take a mental cruise somewhere, but it is adamant about that sort of frivolity. One thing at a time, aphasic, just one!

When physical therapy was begun in the hospital the stroke must have been a week old. The therapist pushed and pulled my leg and arm and talked constantly. Ordinarily, that would have amused me but because aphasia was preempting everything else, it was impossible to listen to the tales being told and still listen for the haphazardly interspersed directions which brought on a "pay attention." That, in turn, brought forth an inaudible mental "Nuts to you. Give me instructions and hush."

There followed considerable bewilderment until I finally decided to try to turn off all but the directions, which was anything but easy. When I graduated to taking a walk up and down the hall, the therapist chortled to anyone within screaming distance, once or twice a walk, "Look, Ma, no hands."

No wonder the occupational therapist was a most refreshing change: quiet, capable, saying only what was needed. I'm still using an exercise she showed me because it seems to be good for my bursitis bitten shoulders and their cracking concrete.

When I left the hospital, physical therapy was transferred to a center which is a living monument to the work of a blithe spirit. Forever I shall be grateful to the doctor who sent me there, for it was the most wonderful lesson in compassion, and empathy, and that loving determination which badly handicapped people seem to have: that every day will be the time when their friends achieve another goal, a tribute to incandescent beauty.

In that center the therapists had the right mixture of genuine praise, ridiculous banter and loving concern. Mine was a delight: intelligent, bursting with energy, eager to know the latest workable treatments devised, and adept and understanding in the exercises she used, especially when they hurt. They were therapists with radiant, warm personalities. I was able to watch them, because in the very large room where therapy took place, there were times when it wasn't quite my turn, times when hot packs soothed part of me, and times when I bicycled to yon and back by sitting still, and that wasn't too difficult since it involved my bum leg which when told to do something did it until told to stop.

This was a center where patients helped other patients, where the atmosphere was a happy demonstration of do unto others. Physical therapy is important from the standpoint of helping the patient set goals he can reach and in encouraging him when he makes any progress, no matter how slight. It seems salutary for patients in physical rehabilitation to be together in therapy. Such togetherness can act as a catalyst for everyone in that each one's painfully slow progress can be viewed in proper perspective when in this modus operandi.

In my case, more physical progress probably would have been made had as much time been devoted to physical therapy as has been to speech therapy. Since an aphasic seems to have an extremely limited supply of energy, should he not have the right to decide for himself where he is going to spend most of it? Frankly, I do not dwell on the physical tasks that are difficult if not impossible for me to do. My arm and hand are making tortoise improvements month by month. It is doubtful if they will ever be completely recovered.

Understandably, everyone has a different goal. Mine, from the first, has been not to be a parasite, a word with frightful implications, hard for me to remember, and has been known to splurt out not *parasite* but *prostitute*! Is that an aphasic approximation or a Freudian flub? What matters is that, for me, speech therapy meant rebuilding the damaged areas in my world of communication. And this world was far more important to me than the one delineated by abilities which physical therapy attempted to revive.

Additional Rehabilitation Team Members

My own rehabilitation team had two more members, the balance wheels: the speech therapist and my husband, both important enough to merit special discussion. Additional team members may depend on the severity of the aphasia, the patient's stability, his family situation, finances, job, and any condition he might have conducive to or detracting from his recovery. They could be a psychologist, psychiatrist, linguist, social worker or anyone else deemed advisable.

There needs to be someone to pick up the pieces, to gather pertinent information from each discipline, follow the patient's every progress, be the bridge between the patient's family and the rehabilitation team or between members of the team. Who can do this better than a social worker? Social workers should be experts on bits and pieces and how they can be made to fit together.

The role of a social worker may continue after the patient's dismissal from the hospital for the therapies as still in force, and the kinds of adjustments the aphasic makes to normal life conditions become apparent, be they good, bad, or so-so. In this period following a stroke the social worker may be a vital cog in helping the patient and his family find their ways to new varieties of living, and to meet these challenges with a measure of enthusiasm and not deadly pessimism.

Speech Therapy and the Academy Of Aphasia

While aphasia is scarcely a new disorder, is much really known about the many ways it can affect those afflicted? There is an organization called the Academy of Aphasia. It has one hundred members which include speech pathologists, psychologists, linguists, physicians, psychiatrists, neurologists, neurosurgeons, all with sensitive expertise since a great deal of their work is with aphasics.

When these members lecture in the hope of disseminating information which could mean a better understanding of aphasia, they should be listened to with open minds and hearts. The import of the remarks by members of this academy may reveal cogent ideas perhaps never imagined, but do their listeners ingest only as much as suits them? Sadly enough, aphasics are not alone in communication distortions.

The thinking which has earned an individual the plaudits of a membership in the Academy Of Aphasia is the kind of forward thinking needed in directing an effective rehabilitation team. It is the sort of alert intelligence that has examined perceptively the many facets of a stroke patient's predicament. These facets, in all their complexity, must be presented and used if the patient is to be rehabilitated in the broadest, deepest sense.

The patient's rallying point is his speech therapist. But are there enough who have had intelligent training in the peculiarities of aphasia? It is to be earnestly hoped that among today's crop of young people, perceptive and aware, there will be many who can see the challenges in successful working with aphasics. May they insist on the merit of training under teachers who have spent much of their adult lives learning from aphasics the multitudinal pathways by which a patient may reach a happy, workable way of living.

As an aphasic who was in a good climate for rehabilitation, I have a subtle, sickish feeling that speech therapy, and everything it stands for, tends to be shoved aside as a minor key in rehabilitation. It should be the most important factor if the patient's needs are to be met intelligently. Too many of those who should know, and those who don't, are like the handicapped person who said to me, "You mean you had to learn to talk again? That couldn't be hard. Besides, who listens to you anyway?" Aw, c'mon kids, isn't it time to listen to aphasics?

Rehabilitation: The Teamwork Approach

The function of rehabilitation is to insure the return of the patient to his own bailiwick in society with a mental outlook and the physical knowhow to make possible a good and rewarding adjustment. Teamwork, to accomplish this, means the ability and desire to help an aphasic gain enough confidence in himself to enable him to change his goals, to make adjustments he never thought about having to make, and to realign values. This kind of teamwork, in effect, serves as an impetus to boost the patient over peaks which may have seemed insurmountable at first.

It ought to occur to this kind of a team that the more they absorb about aphasia the better will be their understanding of strokes and their multi-varied implications. And the greater will be their aid to an aphasic in becoming a productive member of society within the limits of his post-stroke capabilities. The problems stemming from the interruptions of circuits must be explained intelligently to the team, for unless they know the extent of any particular aphasic's difficulties they cannot hope to achieve the goals they set out to reach.

Wouldn't it be feasible for the one directing the thinking of a rehabilitation team to be a member of the Academy Of Aphasia or have been trained by a member? It is such a waste of time, money and talent to travel on an uncharted course blithely ignoring the very source most likely to have directions.

Teamwork, to be effective, presupposes that each member understands his assignment and that he also understands the project in its totality. A keen understanding of aphasia may one day open doors of the mind we have been passing unnoticed for years, with no speculation on the treasures we might find if we dared to fling them wide. Not necessarily would we have to find a Pandora's box.

Further Observations By One Aphasic

Stroke wings are being added to big hospitals, wings which include expensive equipment, functional desgin and overall beauty. Yet little attention seems to be given to aphasia and to those equipped by training and experience to unlock doors to the rehabilitation of the aphasic. I have a desperate, helpless feeling. How can knowledgeable people be doing this? Do these concerned persons, for they are concerned, honestly believe they are striking back at strokes most effectively? Are they inflexible in their attitude toward change, feeling something is right only when it is in accord with their thinking? Or are they *unaware* of the strides made by a select few in tapping the source wherein lie solutions to many of the mysteries revolving around stroke rehabilitation?

Now I am not addicted to caffeine, nicotine, alcohol, drugs or bad thoughts, and though I seem to be slowly turning to cement, before transmutation marbleizes, please listen. I refuse to be daunted, refuse to see millions spent on stroke rehabilitation when an essential ingredient like speech therapy seems to be ignored. I am pleading with those on rehabilitation teams to look at what they are doing and look at it hard.

How, by the purple of anger, can people think it is necessary for the stroke patient to realign *his* values while, at the same time, they are warming themselves with the security blanket of gems like, "A stroke is always a total personal disaster."

Or, "Her mind is almost gone." Anybody with an I.Q. higher than −10 could see the sparks of intelligence locked in the patient's eyes and then watch the shutters close over them as she encounters one more person speaking in an incomprehensible language she is unable to understand. Heartbreaking to see and one wonders how long she must wait for someone to come with the right key to open the door of her aphasia. May she have an extra room in her head as pleasant as mine.

Or, "He can do it if he wants to. Otherwise, why did he do it yesterday but is unable to today?" That person ought to know that there may be a legitimate reason why the patient could do "it" yesterday but not today. He truly needs to know.

Interestingly, each of those aforementioned sterling statements came from professionals. The patient, if he is surrounded on every side by defeating attitudes, can hardly be expected to snake his uncertain way through such a murky mess of molasses and emerge happy and smiling at the top of a compost heap hardly designed to nurture constructive thoughts.

I deem it my prerogative to scatter about a bit those ideas I have gleaned relating to rehabilitation, ideas which seem very important. Surely it is more astringic, or is it more enlivening, to read the thoughts of someone who has been through the mill than to have ideas come only from learned, objective souls who like switching statistics every old which way, but are not quite as excited about dull human figures who don't push as easily.

Please try to imagine what it means to have aphasia. And ponder these things in your hearts. A wise, unlettered, gnarled, dear old lady once told me, "The greatest people are those with understanding hearts and educated heads."

We are daily thankful for the quirk of fate which sent us to *the* hospital where I enjoyed loving care and intelligent concern, and from which there was a happy send-off into the everyday world. Every aphasic is not as fortunate. They all should be.

Chapters three and four have been very hard chapters to write, hard because it is never easy to relive shattering moments. These were moments when I had to examine myself minutely: my weaknesses, my insecurities, my failings as balanced by my strengths, my abilities, my dreams. I had to view all these things tied together by love. I really had to examine me.

If these chapters leave a feeling of being pulled a little this way and twisted a bit that way maybe that is exactly how my encounter with aphasia made me feel. Still, an honest self-appraisal is good catharsis. And, having examined the encounter pretty thoroughly, it is ready to be shoved back in the can of worms where it can wiggle and mold in peace.

I think I needn't look back any more. I'd much rather take a pleasant wonderful walk through the miracles of speech therapy.

5

My Life-Line To Sanity

The Marvels of Speech Therapy

The door opened quietly and then I knew. No words told me that this was the one I needed so badly — a radiant smile did that, and the weights of uncertainty that seemed to be sitting all over me flowed, like mercury, into one great big ball, rolled off and vanished never to return again.

And this was the first miracle speech therapy wrought for me. No word was needed — it was in the magic of a look — an instantaneous rapport partly because my innermost messenger had told me it would be that way. Speech therapy's rare talent is this: being able to hop on anybody's wave length and stay there until the aphasic has learned how to climb the unending tortuous crag facing him.

This therapy develops a facility for relating to seriously ill patients who are trying to remember how to say anything, only by the time they think they may have found out they no longer remember what it was they had set out to discover. And then a therapist comes, a person who knows! And those dreadful empty spaces are of very little moment.

That awful feeling of being a prisoner within myself! How could there be a rote, dispassionate, scientific discussion of what speech therapy can do for an aphasic, for aphasia is not a plain vanilla kind of disorder to which rules 1, 2 and 3 apply and that's it!

A successful therapist has to be intuitively perceptive, attuned to using every clue, things nobody else would suspect were clues; a mind imaginatively sensitive to our needs, wants, desires, frustrations, weariness, hopes, abilities and our obvious disabilities. There must be finesse with words to secure necessary information and patients never need to feel insecure with a therapist. How could they, bolstered as they are by lovely smiles, sweet talk when needed (which is nearly all the time), and genuine encouragement.

Two years post-stroke and I can still feel the indescribable relief when a rescuing therapist opened the door. There seemed to be a golden thread linking us, mind to mind, and I knew that this bit of gossamer gold was my means of getting thinking reorganized; of finding, in my bashed brain, new pathways to trot over or old ones to plod through. This was my life-line to sanity.

What *is* speech therapy? For me, it meant that the therapist would help me find my way back to a degree of normalcy in every single endeavor that required using my mind as it struggled for new strategies in getting thoughts through a damaged brain to the world outside. Who else could there be able to give this kind of necessary assistance?

Isn't that a sizeable order for the therapist and the patient? Not if it concerns aphasia where being able to talk is only one portion of what therapy is structured to do, at least theoretically. Aphasia involves a brain in which the areas of communication have suffered power failures with lines twisted and tangled or so ruined they can never be retrieved. Consequently, therapy is concerned with talking, reading, writing, arithmetic, thinking, doing — all of it leading to the patient's regaining confidence in himself.

Therapy is probably accomplished with the greatest ease when both the therapist and the patient enjoy challenges demanding the best they have to give. Learning has always been fun, so digging in and doing those things which had to be done did not pose a problem with me. While completely immersed in the exhausting task of finding words and trying to say them, I felt only elation over the minutest progress.

How is that feeling of triumph effected? An aphasic needs a sense of humor as much as anything and, hopefully, his therapist approaches with a light touch the many comic/tragic components lacing aphasia. The patient needs a therapist who is not jaded by these wearing experiences, who has a continuing compassionate interest in him, an enthusiasm that never fails and a control that never falters.

One lesson every stroke patient must learn is that therapy never stops. Oh, a therapist may not be needed forever, but the aphasic must continue therapy for the rest of his life if he is to maintain the progress that has been made and make any additional progress deemed possible.

The aphasic's attitude and outlook are vital and imperative factors in his rehabilitation. He cannot set daily goals encompassing too many things to be done, for fatigue is liable to swat him down often, and that day may pass with nothing being finished that he was determined to do. Oh, I'm an old hand at this game, and there is no way of winning it without acceding to the stringent demands aphasia imposes on its chosen victims. So, therapy, while a constant must, needs to be done within the limits each aphasic determines are his.

Pacing himself is a requirement if he is to function reasonably well. When fatigue, that bug-a-boo almost every aphasic lives with, kerplunks right in the midst of everything, the aphasic better stop whatever he is doing, because from that point on nothing will come out properly, his thinker won't think and he needs to change activities or float away in a renewing nap.

This is a lesson that seems to have to be learned anew by me since I'm always sure that this time will be different and really it isn't. It is, also, a lesson that is apparently hard for others to comprehend. Fatigue comes quickly and totally to me after the least little bit of exertion.

Getting directions through a stroke-damaged brain takes tremendous effort. Concentration can be achieved for such a minute period of time and trying to maintain it becomes so difficult that it is hard to realize a simple mental process can provoke a tiredness as acute as this — weariness so complete one can only succumb to it and what if nothing else ever functions again? Does it really make even a dabble of difference? That is the fatigue of my aphasia.

My experience has been that the speech therapist was the only person aware of the totality of fatigue I felt — the only person on whom I could pin my hope for understanding what made me tick. Patients quickly know that the speech therapist is someone to whom they can relate because he has already related to them; that they can count on his interest and his willingness and ability to accept them as part of the human race despite aphasia.

It might be said that I had unrealistic ideas on what speech therapy was going to achieve. Perhaps therapy is not always set up to accomplish what it did for me, or is it rather that what the patient receives may be in proportion to the effort he makes? True, at least in some cases.

Areas Where Speech Therapy Helped Me

The teaching techniques of speech therapy I don't pretend to know anything about — what their results were are tangible. Speech therapy was effective in helping me regain the following facilities in communication:

> talking
> reading
> writing
> arithmetic
> thinking
> post-stroke activities

Talking

Can you imagine discovering that something dreadful had happened to your speech and then being asked to say "Methodist Episcopal"? Wouldn't you like to know how it sounded? I would. That little bit of probing preceded speech therapy and how badly I wanted the therapist. Those two words are still corkers!

No one can know, except an aphasic, what relief the therapist brought and we were actually started on the rocky road to recovery. Not only was there difficulty in finding a word when it was wanted, but it seemed as though the only way it could be captured was in syllables.

While there was bumbling and stumbling and little pieces left way out in the back 40, there was no discouragement, which may seem rather unusual, but that is the way it was. It may have been part of the insulation nature tossed over me, but I suspect that it was mostly the creative climate the therapist wove around me.

For quite a while, though what that meant in terms of definite time, I'm unsure, words being sought continued to arrive in syllables. Usually the root syllable came first and then the puzzle might be solved by working from either end.

One such remembered happening occurred on a day when it would have been so nice if the doctor we have had for nearly twenty-five years could have been there to understand and comfort me. And my thoughts went like this:

"What *is* the word that describes him? . . . . pash . . . . oh, then passion . . . . passion? . . . . good grief! I don't know anything about his passion . . . . that's odd . . . . still, that must be part of the word . . . . now! . . passionate . . . oh, murder! it's getting worse . . . . but I'm sure that's somehow right . . . . ah, finally . . . . compassionate! . . . . . . and so perfect for him . . . . "

By the time the word was rounded up, that seemed sufficient to carry me through another minor crisis dispelling my temporary need of That Very Special Man.

Substitution was a constant solution and isn't it amazing when simple words refuse to come, one can still hunt and scratch and find others — an exhausting procedure, but one that often got the job done. For instance, the wanted word was "globe," but nowhere could it be found and after unending searching the substitution was "map in the round." There have been times when substitution was the only way conversations could be handled — fatiguing for me, but wearing, too, for those listening.

Sometimes words were found in funny little places called "the back way." If the sentence I was trying to say was, "I'll wear a blue dress," which refused to jell, then the back way detour became, "My husband likes to find me in blue."

Unbelievable, that the detours can seem harder than going the quieter original route. Unbelievable, too, how much circumlocution, backtracking, and beginning again can be involved in finishing a simple sentence. Mental acrobatics were used to find a word, or a substitute, without losing the thought — more time and effort than could ever be imagined. Sometimes nothing would come and for the moment it was dropped, then returned to with success.

For me, an important means of regaining a lost ability was to plow ahead and practice, no matter how garbled were the beginning results. It must have seemed to the therapist that I was never going to progress beyond the word "no," for with every word attempted, but wrong, there would come an understandable "no" . . . . try again . . . . "no" . . . . and again and again, until the right word came or a substitute was located or the whole mess forgotten for the time being, while we went on to another something where success was fairly certain. An excellent teaching tool? An excellent strategy to use with anyone having trouble succeeding at anything.

And so it was learned that to maintain any progress in a facility being recouped, I had to continue to use my voice, find pathways and plod over them often enough to make them visible to thoughts sent from my mind and less likely to be erased from lack of trodding. Talking meant just doing it, monitoring, if possible, the mistake made and correcting them on the spot, which meant that often talking was correcting one error after another.

Now, the mistakes are not as prevalent as they were, though there are still plenty and, while my monitor is usually on duty, there are too many times when fatigue whispers, "Don't pay any attention to him," and I don't. Errors are not different from those made in the beginning — just not quite as many of them, as per these:

stroke	spoken as	stock
frost		frog
metaphor		metaflor
dishwasher		dishworship
algae		allergy
excuse		decuse
asked	slurped as	ast
enrich		enrish

Multisyllabic words are apt to run together in their hurry to be said and one quaint appellative is "groceries" — it almost has to be pronounced letter by letter, if anyone could do that with "groceries."

Rapid talk, for whatever reasons, is an impossibility. My thinker doesn't sort out things in their proper sequence fast enough to be jammed through an ailing brain, and my tongue doesn't seem to be able to untie itself easily. Have you ever heard a more sensible explanation than this? Talking *is* tiring and if done too much at a time muscles controlling speech get very uppity and scream at me, "We're not gonna struggle thru one more word."

Their reaction to a few other things is also rebellious: laughing, singing and reading anything aloud. Laughing sounds as though I were having a wild, noisy attack of some kind; singing, formerly confined to the bathtub, can now be used only to frighten people, never on key, tune mislaid, quakery screeches usual; and anything to be read aloud sounds as though I had been running for an hour, voice is palsy-shaky, and there is almost no expression. It's absolutely horrendous!

One day, while waiting for the therapist, the judge and jury in my head decided their prisoner ought to attempt to recite the alphabet. Wowie! I bogged down badly after g, slipped and slushed but ended in triumph with x-y-z. Nothing daunted, I then decided to try it backwards. Lest this sounds insane, a story should make it more plausible.

Once, in the third grade, this then-child was indulging in some abominable behavior distracting the class and annoying the teacher. The punishment for this long-forgotten wickedness was learning the alphabet backwards, but it could hardly have been called punishment — keeping the imp busy and out of mischief, yes. The alphabet was learned backwards and recited and repeated often enough for my own edification that it was never completely mislaid, and even I could say it with the only bobble over w-v-u. One does not know what surprises aphasia offers!

Poky response is one. On a recent day we were going somewhere in the car and I was clutching the letters, which *had* to be mailed in a certain spot. We neared the proper mail box but didn't slow down and when strange signals were sent to Hans he thought they were being waggled to an unknown character we had passed. That's typical for me — nothing comes or if something does it is apt to be jargon. My brain simply will not transmit words in a hurry, so I can't respond to a crisis situation by uttering anything — not even a yell!

There are advantages in talking to oneself, a device to determine where mistakes are being made, what are being used as fill-in words, beyond what speed talking becomes a mush of nothing. Fill-in words are interesting, especially important for aphasics because we are wont to have gaps in conversations when we can't think of words or have forgotten what was being bandied about.

That monster, whose civilized name is 'the telephone'

provides one of the greatest outlets for fill-in words for me — listen . . . well . . . uh . . . ah . . . oh . . . . really . . . . . Since this speed talker of yore has changed to a quiet listener she has heard many oddities: jillions of words meaning absolutely nothing, but wearing in a frenzied sort of way; questions asked but no answers wanted for the speaker wishes to hear only his own opinions; fill-in words that are so rampant one wonders if that is all the conversation involves. (How about "you know" in the middle of nowhere. It makes me cringe to hear me say it.)

Telephoning is a frantic, fearful kind of task, friendly calls excluded, and one has to be ready with any and all information. "They" want (or is it demand) everything: birthdate and hour, social security number, internal revenue status and to heck with my own internals, numbers on the charge plate, auto license, voter registration, American Express and do we tithe?

Never say that ordering a simple casserole dish for a wedding present is easy.

Recently, I tried it again with every bit of information imaginable spread out around me on the bed, the only spot big enough to hold it all. Dialed the number, which was right for a change, and after announcing my request, was switched to someone more efficient. This happened three times over a casserole until I didn't remember the reason for the call. When the third saleslady was ready to become irritated, the trump card was played, and she was told her patience was appreciated for she was speaking to me, a stroke victim.

It helps, upon occasion, to be a Pitiful Pearl. Then came the final blow, for the bit of information the salesperson wanted flew out of my mind, "and what is your phone number?" No idea! But in walked my mate, the rescue was at hand, the casserole has been delivered. Joy to the world!

It is incredible the amount of maneuvering that is required for me to have words come out as they should. I wish I could explain to you how it seems. It is like a computer that has short-circuited but has to be used as it is, manipulations must be made in round-about ways, use any part not in trouble and improvise the rest of the steps. It can be weird.

Aphasia teaches much. It has taught me that talking *can* be accomplished, but it is not the easy, unconscious flowing it was — rather, it is a stilted, deliberate thinking of words. It can be exhausting and it can't be done fast. There are so many ideas, all hurrying to be said. The thought is put in a slot but it won't fit, so another slot has to be tried, and then when it is ready to emerge it must be shoved this way or that to pop out right. Even thoughts get impatient when the brain balks at transmitting them.

It is maddening to have interesting things to say which sound so well in my head, but when said aloud are a mess of slop. One who is eager to help an aphasic must be willing to listen, calm in his approach because he honestly wants to know what the aphasic is trying to tell him. And he doesn't jump pronto to any conclusions.

Aphasia has taught me, too, that talking can be expected to be worse at night when everything about me is tired, and in crowds of people it may be taboo for it means that conversations cannot be differentiated, my voice can't be heard, so there is just one thing to do: resort to mental sassy retorts. They please me, if no one else, and there really is much pleasure in silence.

Reading

It did not occur to me there could be any difficulty with reading, which is probably just as well because words have been, for me, a sustenance of life. It has been such fun to find words that fit into a lovely mosaic — lilting words flowing into a cadence of beauty — funny words adding a dollop of humor to a thought — solemn words fortifying serious ideas — jig saw puzzles of words limitless in their scope and definition and pleasure.

No trouble with reading was clouding the horizon. The work book the therapist brought me — the kind a secretary uses for dictation and easy to handle — had brief, easy to read instructions, one to a page posing no particular problem in ascertaining what those few words meant. Then one day — the exact date naturally escapes me though it was during the first month — a newspaper was brought for me to tackle.

This brings up a moot point: reading was so much a part of me that, if there was nothing of vital interest on hand, my attention would be riveted to signs waving from bill boards or labels on cans. But since the stroke there had not been one request for anything to read.

Did I not know how to ask for a book or which one to mention or could it be that my loving family had asked me and been given a negative answer? Was it drowning fatigue? Or had a clue been brought to me by the cards and notes which were delightful to have, but were proving to be more than I could cope with just then. Reading was too much if there were more than a few words and the things said to me were apt to be overwhelming. But how much did the real reasons for my glancing at the cards and then putting them away for later perusal register except superficially?

Here was the paper! What in the world was I to do with anything as big and cumbersome as a newspaper? And all those words! An article was tackled only to find that all the words were a complete jumble of letters signifying nothing! What a horrible sensation — still no panic. The therapist would help me up and out of this mess. Do all aphasics depend so absolutely on the therapist for help in any area of communication?

As an aid, a short article was found with short paragraphs and it was cut out, which meant no clumsy paper to keep intact in front of me and no extra words to distract me from the reading at hand. The return journey was begun. If a sentence was not long, it was hoped the thought would make sense when the sentence ended. If the paragraph was a small one, maybe its contained thought would be apparent to me. Maybe not. Mastering even the tiniest article took consistent plodding.

Day by day, bit by bit, progress was made. The newspaper is still too busy and while it once was devoured in toto, now days may pass when my attention to the papers is merely a glance at the headlines. It has to be read spread out on a table, and even so what is read is extremely selective. And why not! Perhaps my mind had accumulated too much detritus over the years and rebels at being a trash can.

It is startling how tremendously fatiguing reading can be; my intense, encompassing pleasure has to be indulged in circumspectly. Other reasons for battling this kind of fatigue were known to me, for our two sons were beset with this weariness which I offset by reading to them constantly. Now the great effort reading causes many aphasics is known to me even more intimately.

The subject of the reading material is not as important as its format and the size of the printing. Right now, I am deep in a thoroughly interesting and valuable book, but because of small print it is taking me forever. To my knowledge, it is the only print available, the sort of book which, pre-stroke, would have been read as fast as possible and then reread carefully. Now, it is hard to retain the thought in between readings and if several pages are perused at a sitting, to say nothing of being digested, that is good under current circumstances.

For practice in reading and speaking the *National Geographic* was read aloud every day. It was chosen because it is easy to hold, has beautiful photography and might give me some great tuck-away bits of information. Vain Hope! With a voice devoid of expression no one could have told if I were reading a tome on chemistry, a story with hilarious comedy, or an Aesop's Fable. Literally, almost nothing of the wonders being explored was absorbed by me, apparently reading in an ununderstandable language.

The one-thing-at-a-time lesson aphasia claps atop the victim, me, was being strictly enforced at these reading sessions. If reading was to be done out loud that was enough. Reading and understanding were two things, but only one could be done. My monitor was fairly stern about picking up errors and my efforts produced gems like these:

Dutch Guiana	*read as*	Gutch Duiana
rarely feels		farely reels
ruled Rome		roled Rume
Knights of Malta		Malts of Knighta
spaghetti		scubetti
ground-hugging		hug-grounding
cloud seeding		soud cleeding
surface		circus
Danube		Dabune
bureaucrats		bureaucracks
Capri		Pacri
Blue Grotto		Brue Glotto

Errors being made now have this touch of interest: they are mistakes in silent reading. It must be that those errors are detected because they sound odd or make no sense. For example:

five miles of	*read as*	five pastures of
green pastures		green miles
loved talking		talked lovingly
set the pace		sace the pet

Normal people make lots of funny errors, but when one has been slugged by aphasia he may be more conscious of many of his mistakes, once the monitor starts his obligations. Mine is busy, but he does not always get attention. Oh, he is listened to, if only detachedly, though corrections may not be forthcoming if it is a tired day. On such a day my monitor sleeps fitfully.

Contact with my business partner, when the road calls him, is via the telephone at night and often that leads to rather strange statements from me. There are numbers of letters and bulletins to be read to him, and reading aloud carries with it many chances for aberrations. When words escape me, my entire conversation may be a series of substitutions and in-the-back-way ruses, so that the listener is a little confused, if not bemused, and the informant is as limp as an old soppy rag.

But, there are compensations! One was a going-home gift which arrived upon a lovely day: a book for an aphasic who loves the sound and feeling and flavor of words. It was James Lipton's *An Exaltation of Larks* meant for one who delights in charming combinations of words appealing to one's sense of risibility in delicious quantities. What a marvelous boost for me, for whom it was a perfect gift, a soothing balm for an ego that had been pricked but had not suffered complete deflating.

Writing

It would be nice to have tuppence to give to stroke research for every time this question has been posed, "How long did it take you to learn to write with your left hand?" Inasmuch as my right hand did nothing but vegetate, it seemed easier to use the fingers of my left hand than the toes of my left foot. It was a dilemma not worth wasting time thinking about, so it wasn't ever a dilemma.

When the therapist brought the first work book, there was no "can you," "will you" or "pretty please" — just a realistic assessment of the situation and a firm "here are the tools, let's get busy." And we did.

Never will a certificate for excellence in penmanship be given to me, but the writing is usually legible though the spelling may be strange — *especially* apt to be spelled *escepially* and just the other day *shoved aside* was written *shavide*.

There is a comparison that could be enlightening: it is much easier for me to remember a thought long enough to type it, where in writing the gist of the thought may have flown the coop before the writing is well under way. With me this was not always true.

Now, following a stroke, remembering an idea is a precarious feat. It must be committed to paper immediately, typed if possible, for in the writing it may vanish. Those thoughts that come when lying down for a nap or after going to bed have to be jotted down somehow or they are gone. Thoughts may return, but not as they once did with little persuasion; now they float away mercurially and retrieving them is a maddening procedure.

Spelling can pose a problem that may become a comedy of errors. It was not bothersome pre-stroke in that the guard attending to that area seemed to know when something was amiss and notified me. Now, there are dictionaries everywhere this gal is wont to light. I'm simply unsure about spelling and some days it does seem as though those faithful volumes are being consulted every word or two. Funniest of all is the word that zips through my mind, the very word being hunted, but what in the world does it start with and how is it spelled?

If that seems impossible, it is not, for it has happened too many times with me. How can a word be known to be the right one wanted and yet there is no clear picture in my head of the spelling ? Recently, the word was *jocose*, and for some unknown reason, I thought it began with *k*, which may have been because the *c* in *jocose* sounds like *k* or maybe it was an association in meaning to *knave*.

The k's were perused, though unfruitfully, then the thesaurus was consulted but still the k's brought me no nearer to the object of the search. Finally, *humor* struck a bell, the thesaurus was prodded again, and voila! the puzzle was solved. Hours, literally, have been spent on such detective work but they have not been wasted hours for it is good to feel delight in accomplishment.

Most of the time spelling errors can be caught without much trouble. *Began* may be transposed as *ceban*, checking later will reveal the oddity and saying the sentence out loud usually solves the difficulty. Sometimes a word will be consciously started with the wrong letter — *g* for *j* or *s* for *c* — and there will be confusion over what is out of step but that, too, will evaporate as signals return to the right track.

These may seem like small errors, but they are important to me because they had never been made pre-stroke in quite the same way; perhaps only another aphasic will know that momentary feeling of being in a total wasteland of ignorance. There are ways to combat that empty sensation: top it with the whipped cream of laughter; know it won't last long, so why panic; keep working, for tenacity and continuing therapy will bring results no matter how limited.

It is best not to make any attempt, in the beginning, to

look at the total picture which was my strategy, but was it a conscious one? My first efforts in writing and speaking seemed to consider only the present tense, a maneuver which may have told the therapist things it didn't tell me, for I never noticed. Taking anything step by step, certainly a happening as crucial as aphasia, means one does not need to be overwhelmed by it in toto, for a little piece at a time is not defeating and gives one genuine encouragement.

Write a Valentine for your
husband

WHAT A Nice VALenTime
I Came To give AGAIN To you!

IT so mucH a TaRT of lover
oF MANY Kisses To you

Im So Mice a VaLEnTine
I came To give AGAIn to you

Feb 24, 1990

Hi love babies:

Guess what! David & Synette had a girl, Kelly, just borned last night.

Thank you for everything. you see that I am O.K.

It will be heavenly when I start writing with my right hand

So I'll be going home soon.

I'm coming along very well.

You ought to hear me talk. It couldn't get any younger name to say anything but young. We just laughed and told Daddy that that meant a I'd a Chinese girl who was born 5000 B.C.

That about all for now

mush much love
Mother

SHE WRITES WITH
HER LEFT HAND
DAVID
IS PROGRESSING VERY NICELY.
HOPE TO TAKE HER HOME
BY WEDNESDAY

Write a blanket letter
which would go to
friends and relatives and
would tell them of
your activities.

Thank you for the lovely, lovely
things you sent and for your
telephone calls.

I'm doing very well.

Now I got a peg leg, but it is coming
along, and soon I won't limp.

My right hand will eventually will as good as new.

And holy cow! You should hear me speak! I'm an Aphasic. I gotta slow down and let those wires get unscrambled.

The gibberish they don't know — It's just simple! I was once a kid in 11th century in Wales.

Keep rooting for me

Lovingly
Helen

A later event that was a happy development was the arrival of an electric typewriter, which seemed to make thinking smoother in being transmitted and that made me less restless and less fatigued. My typing can't be considered fast, but it is amazing how much comes through my addled brain into the fingers of my left hand onto paper, incredibly more than were thoughts hand written.

Regrettably, the papers boasting my first writing efforts were thrown away. They would have to have been seen to realize the initial difficulty in doing anything. The preceding examples from my first work book will show the advancement made in the beginning three weeks of therapy. Do they also show the unbelievable labor they represent: concentration that meant unknown pulling and tugging; trying to slip a word along paths that seemed monstrously damaged; and finally, to feel dazzling triumph when one tiny sentence jelled?

They reveal a successful technique. Using consistent, repetitive strategies in untangling lines of communication, the therapist let me set the pace, used my motivation as a guide and let that carry me along when energy had plumb given out, though enthusiasm refused to buckle under.

Arithmetic

Are you querying, "What does math have to do with speech therapy?" If it is easy to mix up words — *am* for *have* or *be* for *do* — why isn't it just as easy to jumble numbers — *123* for *321* or *3714* for *4713*?

Figures are important in the work to be done for my husband, so it was necessary for me to be able to say and write numbers correctly. Believe me! That is a duty requiring daily doing, and demands more concentration, checking and rechecking than once upon an olden time, for it would be harder on me to have mistakes creeping in now in my status as an aphasic.

The books to be kept are not complicated, but they insist on accuracy and it seems to take me twice as long to do things correctly. It is not possible for me to do the myriad chores that were mine pre-stroke. It would be easy to have too much to do which, in turn, would make even the simplest jobs more than I could cope with gracefully. Tasks have to be weeded out, those not vital to a family's happy functioning should be verboten.

That is exactly the way we are managing. Figures *are* vital, and the therapist helped me learn that they could be handled without throwing me into a terrible tizzy IF other things were dropped. There are daily selling figures to be kept, invoices to be tallied and entered under the correct listing, market week figures to be wrestled with, bills to be paid, bank statements balanced, and numbers read by the ton to my Best Friend over the telephone, a real torture.

Had numbers been scrutinized as soon as words were, they might easily have been the awful mess of unscrambleable figures that words were of letters and they probably would have seemed harder to try to assort into identifiable segments. Fortunately, my husband attended to the figure work until I seemed to be ready for the harness again, and there have been no calamitous errors, just a couple of near flip flops. The numbers to be juggled by me are of a simple nature, an adding machine doing most of the tedious labor, so that this is not the kind of math entailing abstract analysis.

The more checking one does, however slowly, the greater may be his inner glow as confidence returns. When one has been on the receiving end of a blow by aphasia, one realizes how choice are tiny bits of accomplishment, and having a bank statement balance is a great big bit. Each little something well done is to be savored with the happy anticipation that the next step will be up and it will be savored one day too.

Thinking

Does it seem odd to you that there is considerable ease in transmitting a thought from my mind to my fingers onto paper but strenuous effort in helping the same thought muddle its way from my mind to this world as speech? The thought would probably not be recognizable as the same one.

It seems as though typing, which involves my undamaged left hand, makes it possible for an idea to by-pass the brain and trot right out on paper via much traveled paths. But typing only *seems* to make that by-pass because the difference in accomplishment is so great. Are typing and speaking two of the many enigmas of aphasia? Methinks aphasia will always be enigmatic to those of us who have been clouted by it.

Thinking is such a marvelous phenomenon, a delight to scientists, philosophers, and plain aphasics like me. It enables us to do the simple and the complex, the specific and the abstract. It was a peculiar sensation to become aware that my thinking was cloudy in an eerie way — fuzzy, opaque — as if nothing of an earthly nature would ever bother me for translation again. Then the restfulness of an enveloping cocoon was quietly replaced by a subtle awareness that something was amiss, but that if earth still claimed me then I must gather my forces, refuse to be a parasite, and find someone to help me get my thinker percolating once more.

And then one lovely day it happened! The clouds rolled back, the hanging haze dissolved, my thinker clicked, the mind-expanding peak had been scaled, the worst was over!

The worst for me — hard work nudges always. And what was it that produced such a wonderful feeling? It was a conundrum.

How could those funny few words mark a turning point? Mine wasn't even a correct example, but the thought tumbling in my mind was, "Aha, this time go beyond a play on a word to a play on the hidden meaning of that word." And there appeared before me a tantalizing remembrance, the sturdy figure of a small son, regaling us knowingly and positively, albeit unscientifically and ungrammatically with, "A piranha is a fish what eats people."

From such little things, so unobtrusively, are miracles evoked. It was as though the transmitter, bringing the wonders of the mind to the world outside, had suffered a power failure, but now the switch was back on, electricity was humming over the lines, the mental cobwebs were swept away, the bruises to my self-esteem were fading.

Who but a therapist would have used intuitive knowledge to perform, so simply, this feat of restoration? And what a blessing I was helped to recognize the magic in a quixotic play on words. The beginning again of abstract thinking, a lovely, healing moment.

Still, it was only a beginning, a wonderful talisman for that extra room in my head, within calling distance when situations needed that memory to hang onto — when, for instance, it was discovered that there was nothing funny about the cartoons in one of my favorite magazines, *The New Yorker*, nor was there anything comical about "Dennis The Menace" or "Peanuts." Misery in painful stabs!

How does any aphasic manage without a life-line to sanity? The confidence I had in the therapist (or would it be more honest to call it dependence) seemed reasonable to me, for sooner or later those cartoons *would* be funny. Dismiss those disturbing thoughts! Don't even think about being patient! Get busy and WORK!

And that is what I did. Time cannot be pinpointed, but the thinking enabling me to enjoy the rollicking, tongue-in-cheek humor of cartoons returned little by little. The ability to analyze cryptic statements came back slowly and in order to retrieve a facility important to me it was necessary to put forth efforts which outraced energy. Repairable damage, coupled with sufficient motivation, warranted synchronizing my mind and a busted brain with tuning more or less on the same beam and not totally off key.

It is interesting the kinds of strategies an aphasic must use if he is not to be considered an incompetent. When the stroke was new, I was unsure many, many times about things said to me — had they been or hadn't they — a feeling of nebulous obscurity, of brumous confusion. What to do about it? One solution seemed evident, although the key to it hung on remembering, a moot point, and it was that if something had been heard three times, then it really had been heard. How many times that stratagem didn't work it is impossible to say, but that it did work quite a few times is certain.

An aphasic may have yawning gaps in his communication system, but he is a thinking human being. Now the fact that a patient is smiling, is aware of the subject at hand, is nodding his approval does not mean that he will remember one solitary thing about that particular confrontation, nor does it mean that he must be balmy to have forgotten. Certainly he was aware while the incident was happening, but with aphasia the strangest things can occur. *Comme ci, comme ca.*

A quality of aphasia I resent is the one-thing-at-a-time routine which seems to be a requirement for my membership in the club. Just remembering how many things once were done at the same time can produce flopping fatigue, and there are days when no one can be sure whether fistfuls of capillaries are supplying oxygen to "me head" or whether they have dwindled to a cozy pair.

Those are days when even my thinker has gone to bed with a big DO NOT DISTURB sign on that extra room belonging to me. But thinking is exciting, and there are other days when my thinker works overtime — when in the midst of a quiet reverie, words will cascade in lively ripples from my mind, and if not captured in type instanter, it may be too late. They were such right words — why must they evaporate so soon?

Times, too, during a restful pastime of watching squirrels play an acrobatic game of follow-the-leader and seeing butterflies splash color on window sills, when in the middle of nature's matinee a whole word (in the days of syllable hunting) drops from an outer post into my mind, without any difficulty charges clear through my brain and is said by me with no stumbling! The word? *Adjudicate!* Fine word, but would I ever be apt to need it and where would it be then — probably back at the outer post from whence it came.

Aphasia an easily understood disorder? No, a paradoxical assortment of mishmashes, weirdos and believe-it-or-nots.

Post-Stroke Activities

Following the formal therapy program comes a finale: post-stroke activities.

What in the world does a speech therapist have to do with

those? Depends on the therapist and the aphasic. Thanks to mine, I've had a wonderful time. On the day of ending a month as a hospital patient, I met a group of nurses the therapist was instructing in the pixillating peculiarities of aphasia. There were holes in my responses to their questions, but I found substitute words or misplaced syllables with enthusiasm because these were professional people who made my efforts easier. Besides, the therapist was there to haul me out of a chasm.

It was a delightful boost to my ego. If I could be with similar groups and be seen as a happy aphasic perhaps it might help to change attitudes. The spark plug in these ventures was the speech therapist who has constant interest in what would be good for a specific patient, and an innate wisdom in having professionals see and hear an aphasic on the road back — a two way street: good for them and mightily good for me.

There has been writing, too, therapeutic for me and, as in the development of any ability, the more one exercises it by doing it, the better are the results — certainly an important feature to an aphasic who may be more cognizant of his missteps than he ever was before he was zapped.

Summary

You may ask by now, "Do you really think speech therapy is structured to do everything you have told us? You make it sound like a complete rebuilding job. Should it be? The speech therapist for an aphasic must be awfully special!"

Bless all therapists whose forte is aphasia. They *are* unique. Theirs is a healing art used deftly with a disorder whose implications are only now beginning to be understood. Is there any other discipline prepared to secure the same results?

Doesn't one receive from a discipline results in proportion to the effort he gives? The interaction between a therapist and the aphasic is vital in the patient's success in areas where he wishes to achieve. The aphasic may never be able to make much progess in speaking but a sanguine attitude toward the total picture means progress in his revival as an adjusted, functioning person — progress sparked and nurtured by the techniques and perception of the therapist.

One light

glowing thru the mist

One soft light
>   leading ignorance to
>   the radiance of learning
One life-line to sanity.

Pages from My Workbooks

Pages from my work books used in formal therapy are interesting from the points of view of what needed to be accomplished and how it was effected.

Two Weeks Post-Stroke

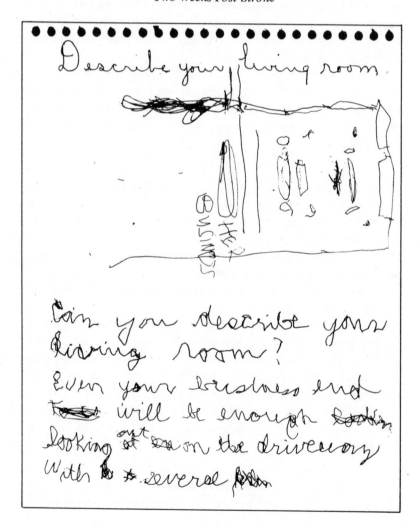

Words that begin with S

Smiley   Slaughter
Santa Claus   Sunlight
Surly   Starlight
Smirched   Sundurn
Star-gazer   Same
Smother   Semi

Words that begin with m

Mangle (3ni 13)   Marbles
Memorabia   Messbine
Memory   Monkey
Mingle   Mind
Mother   Messy
Monks   Mink
Mouse   Mime
Mountain   Marble

Words that rhyme with

love
dove
— haven
— Jove
— mauve
cove
heart
dart
part
tart
Cupid
(?)   Stupid
Cupid   Cupcart
          tulep (sp)

Why do we have policeman?
1. To HeLP us obey tHe LAW
2.

Why do we eat?
1. To KeeP us ALiVe
2.

A A A

automobiles american association

J F K

John Fitzgerald K ennedy

H H W

Hansi (Herman) wanted many

U S A

United States of America

U A W

united american worker

A A U W

association of the american university Women

A A

alcholics anymous

L B J

Lydon Baines Johnson

How is a play different
from a novel?
Plays are written with
directions for both format
and actors.

A novel gives some choices
to as many as the readers
are.

Contractions

I am ~ I'm

I do not ~ I'm not

I will not ~ I'll not

I cannot ~ I can't

I would ~

I will ~ I'll

A Typical Day now

1. 7:15 get up and got a bath
2. 8:00 P. bus was in the parking lot. It had been there all night — whoopse
3. 8:30 W. had breakfast together. —
   and we chatted a whole bunch.
4. Mrs. Wallace did therapy
5. M. What-is-name did more therapy
6. Mrs. Wallace did more therapy
7. I lay down that and try to get rid of that Headache
8. Mrs. Wallace did therapy to bed.

Make up a sentence until
after we ~~sent~~ the help ~~we~~ ~~did just~~ ~~the~~
you ~~asked~~ we to.

(after)

~~He Hums~~ The guest is a great one until after.

until it ~~rained~~, we ~~may~~ were
forced to ~~water~~ ~~that~~ the new tree.

(until)

until after the love-affair
is over, we ~~did~~ as we ~~were~~
were asked.

the

~~He~~ The meadow is fragrant

is

This is a very bright maple.

Write a sentence with :

rite

That is a very meaningful rite of the church.

right   are right or wrong.

It's determine how many things we can be sure.

hair   yuk like mine

Hair can be beautiful and stay put or it can be

hare

pill.
The hare is one creature who never heard of the

peel
The ~~smooth~~ peel of a banana is a
        great to produce sprouted out embarrass-
                                            ment

peal

The peal of the church bell is a gladsome
thing to hear.

How much of a word do
you have to have before you
can recall it? What part
of the word must you have
to have?

Sometimes I don't need any. The words just
pop into my head - as the word adhesive.
I found the word preposition by having "pre"
and the word preparation by having "prep"

Often it seems that words we are unlikely to
use come "whole" - as the word adjudicate.

But the words that are more familiar just escape
us - sometimes they come little by little or after some
thinking they pop - literally

Most of the time if I know the root then eventually I'll
get the word.

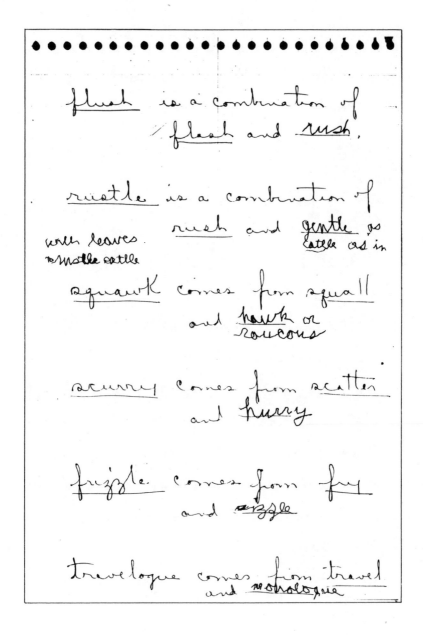

flush is a combination of
flash and rush.

rustle is a combination of
rush and gentle as
with leaves.   cattle as in
rustle cattle

squawk comes from squall
and hawk or
raucous

scurry comes from scatter
and hurry

frizzle comes from fry
and sizzle

travelogue comes from travel
and monologue

With which form of word might
you have difficulty:

    rain   rainy   raining

    part   party   parting

    test   testy   testing

At this point it seems to me I either don't
get the word I want or it comes to me whole.
In conversations I do plenty of substituting
not all of it accurate. For 3 days I've been
hunting the word Capillary. No part of it came
to me, instead of suddenly the whole word.
What I used in a sort of odd way was
pheriphery.

I'll watch more + see if that continues to
happen or if I get part of a word.

86

What do you associate with:

hum   - bees

whistle - Hans

croak - frogs

chirp - crickets

groan - me. getting out of bed when
         nobody's around

chug - train

honk - wild geese

a chica returning to get something about which you
          where have said no. Exasperating
raucous laughter - supposed to be derision but
I don't necessarily hoot - associate it with that.

tinkle . bathroom

why in the world Knock - car is knocking and
                   haven't I noticed it

hiss - snakes. ugh.

bark - Baron

buzz - June bugs trying to
          get in or out .

chatter - a hen session

peep - baby birds or chicks

God has made for us:
Spring day sun-drenched —
  trees gossamer in frothing green —
  or fragrant with blossoms white and pink —
  and jonquils whispering
  world, how beautiful you are.
and babies too,
  the first cry —
    the perfect tiny hand —
    the amazing awareness of everything —
    the all-knowing look —
    the unending questions —
    the dimpled body dappled with the
    sun-kissed rays of hope.
Hope and enthusiasm and
    a sense of humor
and summer's fun.

Sail boats on blue-green water —
and on a warm, lazy day
people fishing and dreaming
and the mourning dove crooning his poignant song.
disappointment past — good things ahead —
Today a blessed hiatus of warmth and beauty
and peace that glows in a secret place.
and when the wind is strong, shadows about —
thunder comes booming —
        and rain strikes savagely.
Wonder to see it is, within a fire-lit room,
Matching our hearts beat
Suddenly its over — The magnificent rainbow
lights the beauty inside of us.
and quietly — so quietly
the leaves have changed the world to color.
        reds and gold
and a time for anticipating.

● ●

We see it on the faces of the very old —   3.
    strength in having lived so long —
    smiles and tears,
    your patience, expectancy, and most of all love.
One starry night the world is full of a
    winter fragrance —
the first snow will come
    pristine in its whiteness
a time for reminiscing —
for discarding things worn out and useless —
a lovely time for beginning anew.
Spring Day sun - drenched
    Trees gossamer in frothing green —
or fragrant with blossoms white and pink —
and jonquils whispering
world — how beautiful you are

• •

6

Me and My Alter Ego

The Import of a Marriage

Have you ever wondered what happens to a marriage when the unruly roomer named Stroke Mit Aphasia moves in with an announced stay of forever and a day? Two weeks, two months, maybe even two years could be managed, but for the rest of the afflicted one's life to have to wrestle with an unwanted, unplanned, unpredictable so-and-such!??!

How is it done? The ways are as numerous as the marriages, an infinite variety among generalities such as these: if the marriage was not built on a firm foundation it may founder; if it has a sturdy foundation but many goals must be realigned and neither partner is eager to adjust, it may be headed for rocky times after an initial acquiescence to shock; if the partners have worked hard over many years to make their marriage a success, then they are apt to consider this one more challenge, find any merits in the new permanent situation, toss out as many demerits as they can feasibly, and adjust to the rest with enthusiasm if not energy. In short, they may find their union has been blessed with an added dimension of tenderness and understanding — even if the aphasic has a terrible time kissing.

Adapting to aphasia is a dilemma for which there are no easy, magic solutions, and when a marriage has been pummeled and bruised by a stroke with aphasia, the needs of both partners have to be examined minutely, carefully, wisely, and with optimistic realism. How can anyone tell, without digging, which marriages will ride the waves made by aphasia and which will drown?

Each marriage is structured quite differently and my assessment of my own is that the foundation for it was laid long before the Man of My Heart appeared. Had my goals differed markedly from his the structure might have zigged where it should have zagged, but since our goals differed only in flavor, not in essentials, we were able to forge a successful merger: the union of a realist and a romanticist.

Quite evident in our marriage are the fruits of our early training and perceptions and almost the incorporating into our own chemistry the qualities and attitudes of our parents. And these are part of the many factors that go into making the secret formula of any marriage — secret because it is doubtful if anyone really knows all the ingredients that are tossed and stirred to make one special concoction for two special people.

The warp and weft of a marriage may be loomed from challenging differences, laced with humor and tolerance and a healthy respect for each other's inherent right to privacy, to thoughts of one's own. If it is lined and overlaid with love, it becomes a firm foundation for a marriage with proportions that are right for the couple involved. And, the stronger a marriage the better chance of adjusting to a bad blow with a minimum of discomfort.

A marriage may look fine from the outside, but is it shored up by the necessities of affection, politeness, joy, laughter, consideration and indispensable humor — all qualities that need to be used in abundance? These are not bestowed by wishing for them — they are gained by thought, an occasional collision, and daily hard work.

As one, we began the marvelous process of learning day by day the strategies enabling two people to recognize the merits of temperamental distinctions; that a union can capture splendor when each partner realizes that those things which bother him may not disturb his mate, so that sort of difference becomes a tool for learning consideration and compromise. We began the continual unfolding of love with its many facets and we came upon the eternally amazing fact that one can be married to one's best friend.

We found marriage a ring, a protective ring, giving us a cushion against the daily onslaughts of ordinary living beyond the circle which enfolded us. Miraculously, the years rushed by almost tripping over each other in their eagerness to reach the next goal . . . and suddenly . . . quietly . . . the impossible accident . . . . All those years of building that marriage served us well.

Striking of a Stroke

Does it seem rather peculiar to be bothered by "parasite" when the stroke was brand new? I had floated through the invisible curtain separating this plane from the next while being held on this plane by my Achilles heel, and my knowing me watched with marked interest the vacillating of this human form. It was curious the anticipation, the ineffable peace, the subdued humming of excitement pervading the part of me that is indestructible . . . . and then the awful denoument when the realization flooded through me that my battered self had to continue to wrestle with terra firma.

I had been on that other side . . . briefly, yes, but long enough to have much shown me, and there was no hurting, ailing body to contend with and no clunky brain either . . . . . yet, here I was still on this earth plane with a hurting, ailing body and a clunky brain. The cosmic link that said "not yet" would help me garner my forces to combat the whatever.

It was a moment when I felt utterly drained of everything positive . . . . . . still on this plane but a nothing which was my horrible concern, for being a nothing was something I could not, would not do to the one I had loved for so many years. How not to bring this crashing down upon him?

And then a pendulum swung back and forth across my mind droning "parasite" . . . . . . "parasite" . . . . . back and forth . . . . . . again and again . . . . . . over and over . . . . . . until "parasite" became "has to be a reason" . . . . . . "has to be a reason" . . . . . . like The Little Engine That Could. So, disappointment was shoved into its customary cubbyhole and the hypnotic droning became the calming busyness of work to be done.

All this time what was happening to My Very Dear? It must have been a shocking experience for him to have seen me, apparently my usual self; to hear a thump and find me crumpled on the bathroom floor; somehow drag my unconscious weight onto my bed; realize I am conscious but communicating only in senseless sounds; make telephone calls — one to a man whose name was dredged from who knows what subterranean cave — and finally get me into a hospital where personnel knew what to do.

Thus went the first day and the second with many tests being made, and during the early evening hours of the second night there was an arteriogram, after which he must have reached the nadir of discouragement. He says he saw it and was told he would have to face one of two alternatives: "Either your wife will die or she will be a vegetable. Oh, there is a remote chance, one you must not count on, but it has happened that some people are born with extra tiny capillaries that will be able to service the damaged side of her brain — a very remote possibility. In twenty-four hours we should know."
..... The exact words we'll never know. We don't even know who told him.

For much of those first few days, my comfit was a carefree insouciance, but what happened to my husband and son remains their private thought, for both are chary of words and since it is now past, so be it. It was comforting to know that My Dear was not alone — one of our children was with him and that one is A Rock, whose name should be *Peter*. Not once did they indicate to me that my obvious illness was anything to cause dreadful concern, which increased my desire for uneventful recovery.

A personal meeting with death is an awing experience. For me, it held the most illuminating, comfortable, peaceful beauty imaginable — a loveliness beyond words. For Hans, it had to be quite different. It was a Something we had not anticipated. We had made plans for the contingency of my being left with our quartet without their father: insurance had been purchased, a mint of it so it seemed; our wills were in order; and we had arranged for the shells of ourselves to be given to a medical school.

Yes, we had planned intellectually, practically. But, . . . emotionally? . . . . . I'm not sure we ever gave much thought to the idea of death coming to either of us. And then the stroke happened and we found out how tenuous are the earthly ties of even a strong marriage. We learned anew the continuing miracle of love; there was fresh meaning to being needed, tapped by the vibrant best of my mate; and I literally plunged into the business of getting well, knowing there was a healing magnetism in having those dearest to me care so much.

Where there is a marriage whose mates have given each other a great deal of latitude and respect and have bestowed the same latitude and respect on their children, lacing the relationships with myriad tendrils of love, a tightly knit family is found. Such is ours. What did it mean? It may have meant the difference between a happy outcome following aphasia or one that might have been muddled.

The stroke couldn't have sat on me at a better time, assuming there is a good time to have one. The last cub was in college away from home which meant no more daily hordes of swarming young people, and it seemed odd that where those were normal events to which I had looked forward and enjoyed, now there was thankfulness to have that activity end. Had the stroke come a year or two earlier it would not have been easy for merry adjustment.

This way there was time for me to recoup part of my losses in blessed privacy, which is not the way every aphasic would like to have it. We have heard and read of aphasics who needed surrounding by people, but my family knew, with me, that strategy would lead to desperation and a straitjacket. Even that might have changed had there been a different or a more severe damage. Doesn't it boil down to how well do those caring for and living with an aphasic know the person, how perceptive are they, how imaginative, and how secure?

Our children have never been impatient or cross with me. There is good to be learned from any disaster that may befall us, and when younger ones are impelled to do those things which were customarily the province of the older ones, perhaps it behooves the older souls to acquiesce gracefully. It is a fine line for both to tread and it surely can be contended that the more secure those involved are, the greater will be the ease of transition.

Let's get back to Mein Mann by now recuperated from the shock he must have been handed knowing his do-it-myself wife had been slugged by a stroke. After his initial poise, how did he act? This aphasic thinks he should be listed in the roster of The Quietly Great.

One of the most therapeutic things Schatze did for me was to go on the trip planned for us both. There were people waiting for him who needed to see him, he didn't have to wonder where I was, our son was on hand, and it would have made me uncomfortable if he hadn't gone. Therapy was beginning, and having him around twiddling his thumbs when he should have been elsewhere was inane. Being busy at his own work would surely be good for him, too.

So he left and each night, when our son arrived at the hospital, we had a call from his Dad. My contribution was an understandable "hello," "fine," and the usual good night bon mot. When he returned, the improvement was sufficient for him to be elated, and that night he stayed in his motor showroom on the hospital parking lot. The next morning we had breakfast together while we gossiped about the people and the business (he talked — I nodded), and then he said he was thinking about a trip we might take when summer came. That was all . . . . . That was enough and very wise.

The one weekend spent at home before being released from the hospital was sufficient to alert M'sieur to the dangers of having too many people around me, for my extremely limited energy could be seen draining away in the midst of confusion, noise, people, and questions. If I were to go to therapy and work on lessons in-between sessions it would have to be done on terms he knew could be tolerated until I was strong enough to set my own terms.

Did anyone really know how difficult it was to do anything? My husband and the speech therapist were aware of the struggle — a struggle there was no way to get ahead of unless I had a defined goal. Anything to be accomplished was set up as a goal for that hour or that morning or that day, but muddying the stream with too many goals became a story of utter frustration. And I found myself re-learning over and again one of the fateful consequences of my aphasia: think of, plan for, and do only one thing at a time . . . just one.

When one is as loaded with energy as my Alter Ego, it is amazing to find him perceptive and understanding of my limitations and to manage so astutely his aphasic wife. Even though I had never been able to keep up with him in the energy department, he had not seen me with such a minuscule amount. He has known what to do. Give him stars by the boxful — medals by the ton!

The day I came home to stay he gave me a lovely present: our house to myself for several hours. It was a beautiful expectant day — frothy trees, flowers budding in early spring raiment, birds thanking the the sun for shining, the breeze rippling the lake and making music everywhere it went. And when he was safely gone, I got up to wander through every room — some bright with sunshine, some resting from the morning's sunny activities.

It was then, for the first time since the stroke, the deep-down realization coursed through me that vacillation was not my cup of tea — I was here to stay; that it was wisest not to slip too often into the comforting loveliness of an aura I couldn't know completely while earth bound; and although it was early, I knew that writing would be my best mode of communication. So, my life was picked up again where it had been dropped, but it was to be quite a different kind of life.

Common Sense Approach to: Problem Areas

Things have been remarkably smooth although there have been a few moments when everything has gone wrong, when aphasia compounded by fatigue makes an explanation an impossibility, when utter frustration may lead to a severe headache and internal upsets such as have never been experienced. No one needs to tell me I've been working too hard. I know that. Know why too. Know I must be alone until the bad time is at an end. Most of these unglued moments happen when I'm by myself anyway and nobody needs to know about them.

Twice — no one could call that very many — my Traveling Man called to find me in the middle of a session of misery and, of course, the call came at night, not a good telephone hour for me. Both times he knew what had caused the upheaval but it was upsetting to him because he wasn't on hand to "make it all better," and it was upsetting to me for having so little control.

These are uncomfortable moments for it is disheartening having many things I'm eager to do but stamina and ability unequal to the demands. My Dear is aware of such times, knows why they happen, has learned what will prevent them, and usually is calm about them. These are moments when a sense of humor is a required palliative no matter how impossible that may seem. Mein Mann *has* to wear it. His Frau *ought* to.

These unhappy times have never been severe enough to

strain the seams of our marriage, perhaps because those seams have never been bulged to bursting and the discouraging times have been rare. If it seems odd to my husband knowing my adjustability factor sometimes has been lowered close to the zero mark, he does not act as though aphasia is a pretty crummy box of tricks to have dumped on us. Happily and gratefully, he handles me always with a smile and a great big bit of T.L.C.

The happy banter that is a part of our family merriment has not stopped, not even when the stroke was new. Can't most of us tell by the expression in eyes whether someone has understood or if confusion reigns, and what wonderful therapy to have those nearest and dearest to a patient with aphasia show no change in their behavior toward him.

The children delight in having me entertain them and, upon occasion, their friends, by pronouncing such bloopers as *appreciate, social security* and *groceries*. After one very funny session, a friend innocently inquired, "What kind of an accent does your mother have?" . . . . "Do you mean where was she born?" . . . . "Uh huh" . . . . "Up North" . . . . "Gollee, do northerners talk like that?" . . . . Lest you are worried, compatriots, truth will out.

We have been most fortunate. The adjustments we have made because of my stroke have been minimal for a variety of reasons: the aphasia was repairable; speech therapy was begun a week after the stroke; my family never acted as though anything catastrophic was happening; learning is fun to me and I rejoiced in the tiniest improvement, thought the mistakes I made were pretty funny, and plowed ahead confident that there would come a better day.

Although I may never be able to speak with the ease of once upon a long time ago, it was not required of me to face an inevitable fact confronting too many aphasics, that they can never regain their before stroke abilities in the area of communication. For Hans and me, our backgrounds, training, education, maybe whatever body chemistry we were endowed with, and certainly good fortune, helped us meet the situation squarely, and we were grateful for its intrinsic merits, knowing full well that it might easily have been otherwise.

One of the main assets in our ease of adjustment is my husband's work necessitating travel. These times, away from each other, have been renewing. Among other things, it has meant that he could see the progress I was making, which is hard to evaluate if one is never away from the situation, and this gave us both a welcome dollop of encouragement.

We have found that a marriage built on apartness has subtle assets. Some couples do not thrive on togetherness in patches, but for us it has kept being wed sprinkled with the flavor of freshness, and the twist of aphasia has strengthened these imperatives of every marriage: using one's best manners at home; the effectiveness of affection, its need and demonstration; the reviving power of joy.

It was most important to me as an aphasic and to us as a team that we make the jigsaw puzzle of living rewarding. We learned early in our life together that it was possible not to agree without getting tearing mad, so we never have had problems causing anything more than momentary discomfiture. We were adaptable enough to make any disagreement easily solved and always there was the refreshment of time away from each other, time when we could realign our sights, laugh at ourselves, see another viewpoint, and be eager for the next happy home-again.

That Dear of mine has run interference for me at every turn when he is home; he has learned to gauge what I can do and when a halt should be called; he plans activities and trips he feels sure can be handled; he encourages me in endeavors he knows are important to me; he propels me in areas where enthusiasm is not at its highest, such as making an involved phone call. With my mate in charge I'm willing to do things he deems possible. Without him, I might become a recluse.

In essence, our problem solving since aphasia has been more in the nature of problem prevention. We are most thankful that timing has been good, for, with the youngest of our children almost beyond our jurisdiction, we are reaching the savoring period when we are free to enjoy each other without having so many tentacles of responsibility pulling us in diverse directions at any given moment. It is a freedom enhanced by tranquility.

Business Routines

Common sense and our feeling for each other have enabled us to view even icky situations in perspective. For example, when the stroke took me out of circulation, Himself lost his Girl Friday. But he is a realist without one ounce of self-pity. He could have felt guilty as he kept unearthing more and more jobs customarily done by me. Or he could have punished me for having the temerity to have a disabling stroke.

Some people, regrettably, never mature emotionally beyond the infantile anger often felt by children when a mother is seriously ill or has died. Then they vent their hostility smack dab on her by thinking she has done "this" to them deliberately. Nor are children the only ones who act thusly.

What of the Girl Friday? I could have been outraged by thinking the stroke was all *his* fault for expecting me to do so much and I could have punished him forever and a day by never letting him forget it. There are some silly goons who inflict this damaging treatment on each other for much lesser reasons than aphasia. Doesn't an uneventful recovery depend, in part, on the foundation two people have used in building their marriage? It certainly depends on their love for each other and their adaptability.

For some months following the stroke — how many there were we are unsure — Hans paid all the bills. This was a chore he was unused to and a revelation which must have been disconcerting in spots though he rarely said much. Methinks he may have lowered the boom on a couple of the principal offenders but everyone was careful not to bother me about it.

Then, for another period of time, he signed bundles of checks and let me make them out. One happy day, when I was considerably surer of my writing, our banks accepted signatures made with both hands and the bill paying now belongs to me again. Checks are made out with my left hand and signed with my right, a laborious task, but there are days when my signature looks almost normal. There are times when it more than faintly resembles drunken flip-flops.

My work as our office manager poses a problem we have not as yet solved to our mutual satisfaction. Our solutions have been temporary, makeshift ones. I have a feeling that in the beginning, when the stroke was new, my thinking, and perhaps his, was that it wouldn't be too awfully long before things would be manageable again. Then it became "maybe some time." Now it is "probably never."

My candid opinion is that our office, which I would have to get to and from on my own, is off limits. Nor can we overlook a rather numbing fact that people are very enervating. Selling our lines between markets, working the customary market weeks stints, keeping our office in order are — let's face it — beyond my energy output and my abilities, trussed up as I am with one halting arm, one inconsiderate leg, and the limping leftovers of aphasia.

The behind-the-scene work with orders, invoices, and records was done at first by nobody. Then I devised a great scheme we had never used before. Those orders and invoices are still sitting in their clunky files ready for the discard heap, though they weren't a total loss by any means. Anything that kept me THAT busy had to be therapy of some sort. Then some of our faithful helpers checked what we deemed necessary. These might be called searching solutions.

For the present, orders, invoices, and records are attended to by me, slow to be sure, but they are up to date and they are taken care of at home. One office procedure, unattended since the stroke swatted me, involves a cardex system of all our customers — not a vital step but one statistically valuable.

We have a prize assistant who attends to customers between markets, but manning the showroom on a regular basis is unworkable for her. There are many ideas buzzing in our heads and time will tell which one we'll work on next. For the nonce, disasters are in abeyance and everything that has to be done is right on target.

Most situations are not insurmountable. If one uses common sense and compromise, employs whatever can be salvaged no matter how limited that may be, and flavors the whole thing with imagination, solutions can be found that warrant trying even for a little while. Here again, the adaptability of both partners is of prime import. For one thing, it means using a realistic, optimistic approach to any problem without discarding basic values.

Kitchen Play

Meal-getting is an area in which we could be having problems *if* my marriage partner knew nothing about kitchen life. Oh, how lucky I am! He can cook anything and has fun doing it. Actually, he takes over most of the cooking when he is home; takes me lots of places for dinner, which is enjoyed if we are not surrounded by people who seem to be everywhere crawling and shouting.

Occasionally, Myself will fix a roast and all the trimmings, which means that the potatoes, carrots, onions, and whatnot must be

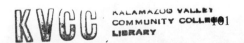

deftly removed from a hot roaster, my boob hand watched so it doesn't get another bad burn, the gravy made with the pan sliding precariously. But why name all the hazards? Need I mention that such a feat can be a frazzling experience since there are too many things to be done nearly simultaneously, and I am still quite close to the one-thing-at-a-time routine which has dogged me consistently in the wake of the stroke.

There are a variety of edibles not demanding hot pans, hot food, and both hands. For instance, I am adept at hard-boiling eggs. Too many burns, and trying to mesh timing with quickness and agility nix cooking eggs any other way. Those who have a yen for them a fraction over three minutes – nothing more or less – can jolly well fix their own. And so it goes. No need to bore you with more.

It is possible for me to go to the grocery store but it is not one of my favorite occupations, for a supermarket can be a confusing, exhausting place to locate needs or luxuries. It used to be a wonder of variety, a delight in planning ahead, an interesting view of wares and people. Now that necessary stint is handled best if a list is made out and the shopping done by some of the children or their father.

Even the nicest meals are kept simple and, despite the foregoing which might be read as a meal mess, I enjoy having company for lunch or dinner. That is much more fun than dining out when I may miss most of the conversation, and what a wonderful, happy lift to have those most dear to me in my own home.

Housekeeping Chores

There is the perennial problem of keeping house. Overlooking the fact that cleaning house is one of the few things I simply detest, one has to admit it isn't exactly a one-handed cinch. My one helper, and the only one I want since she needs no instructions, can come just occasionally. It is truly a blessing for us all that none of us has been used to a compulsive housekeeper and straightener upper.

Also, as if to reinforce the above iffyness, there is a situation which might have led to unmitigated double q jasper had we not taken our usual realistic approach to the mess: we have closed doors and shut our eyes to the conglomerate disorder.

The situation is that as the year 1970 dawned, we had plans for executing a monumental job of redecorating, a feat that hadn't been accomplished since a complete renovation too many years ago. We had lovely plans. The stroke not only damaged my brain, it ruined the plans.

It also brought forth this philosophy: what we did about the impact of the stroke on our viable lives was our prime concern; what happened to the plans was an unimportant consequence. And that attitude could account for our adaptability.

We live in our den-dining-kitchen area, our bedroom and bath, conveniently all close. And while these rooms are piled high with books, business stuff, my inspiration corner with typewriter, paper, letters, and mementoes every whichwhere, I can usually keep these rooms reasonably clean, though it must be admitted we always look like a potpourri of stirred up living.

Business details and writing can be managed by me at my own speed in my own way. But no longer can I supervise workmen, give directions, make instant decisions about little nothings — Where shall we put these? How high should that be? Is this color right? Oh woe is me! All that plus waiting for them to come, and champing at the bit for them to go.

Methinks decision making better bypass me for, where they were no problem, I find decisions unbelievably difficult. Maybe I'm just plain tired of making so many of them and aphasia becomes an excuse. Perhaps the real clinker is that lots of decisions go hand-in-hand with instructions which means getting ideas through my dented brain and told to somebody. Horrors! That's double jeopardy! Whatever the reasons, decisions are a gadfly bother.

I have been on a pretty even keel ever since the stroke bopped me, but we know that I cannot be surrounded by people. The things that I can do are important to us both, and our decision not to renovate, until there is enough time for my husband to begin and finish overseeing the redecoration, was surely wiser.

My Dear anticipates many of my needs; he has learned by listening and watching and is realistic enough to know that planning must be around me — the way I am, not the way some book says I should be. Where other people are involved, he is firm about the things he knows I can do and equally firm when they ought to be verboten. This is called avoiding troubles by anticipating them. It is also termed *common sense*.

Sex: Yes or No

The quietly private area of our relationship with each other needs no discussion, nor, frankly, does it belong to anyone but us. However, sex is an area about which there is much speculation and curiosity and, though it boasts an already glutted market, is there a book on Sex After Stroke?

In my position as a handicapped person, though I never think of myself as that, why is my sex life so all fired important to some professionals and any number of the laity?

Surely they do not think that a good, successful marriage depends for its viability solely on fun frolics in bed. Or do they? Odd that some "knowing" people have ideas about sex which they liberally apply to others, but never to themselves. After all, *they* are different. Well, we are too.

Now, marriage should age like wine, and the older it grows, the more pitfalls it has jumped over or skirted, the more peaks it has climbed, the more rain, sleet, and sunshine it has weathered, and the more the partners to this union have matured in loving, in tolerance, in humor, the headier will be the bouquet.

Between a twosome married for several decades loving is found in ways other than the universal one of intercourse. There are signals sent which they alone recognize; there are looks and touches and whispers meant only for each other; and in a happy union there is a subtle communication based on compassionate understanding and tender love. When aphasia has felled one partner there can be an unconscious plea for help, a plea which the mate hopefully recognizes deep in his protoplasm and meets with concerned intelligence.

In anything as devastating as a stroke is purported to be, there aren't any whiz-bang, easy solutions instanter. There are, understandably, different problems for different people.

Sex may be one of them. But doesn't that depend on the severity of the stroke, the status of the marriage at the time of this shattering ailment, the resiliency of the partners and how well the unimpaired mate can cope with a disorder as paradoxical as a stroke and aphasia? It may depend, also, on how defeated the aphasic is and how much of his self-image he has been able to retrieve, which, in turn, revolves around how much he had in the first place.

As an aphasic I have learned that I must live with

incomparable fatigue — a devastating tiredness that can settle over me without notice, quietly, totally. It is now well over two years since the stroke. And there are still too many days when to do anything takes energy which must be recalled from a never-never land. On these suffocatingly weary days how easy it would be to drift into a limbo of nothingness. It takes effort, an over and over again effort, a seemingly impossible mental exercise to say or do anything. And yet, resisting the impulse to drift may be a key to ongoing recovery.

This drowning tiredness, understood by very few, invades every fiber of me, pushing everything into a momentary vacuum. Sex is part of the everything. But even though it may be temporarily verboten, does that mean putting a permanent quietus on that activity? Himself now knows that I won't break.

We continually change imperceptibly and our marriage has a different tempo than when it began. In the beginning our life together was buoyed by the ecstasy of loving each other so much. And then there were years of ordinary trials, problems, happenings, successes, children, worries, failures, sadness, illness, fun, but, in retrospect, every one of these became a remembering of happiness in depth, of misery glossed over by the passage of time. And there were glimpses of beauty unalloyed, of perceptions coming in moments of reflections.

The years zipped by and we found ourselves meandering along a pleasant road in restful, companionable atunement. Suddenly, without warning, the roadway ended in the chasm of aphasia.

We did not fret over inevitable imponderables. We salvaged the best there was. For some aphasics this may mean much; for others very little. It may mean a before-stroke-and-aphasia resumption of sex patterns, or it may mean a diminution of sexual activity, or it may mean its complete cessation.

In any event, living with an aphasic who, in turn, has to manage an unwelcome forever intruder, demands more internal stamina than either partner may have known was available. But, with the discovery of that stamina and the imagination to propel it, we are finding lovely rewards: learning how adaptable we are; pursuing new interests enthusiastically; finding new friends; and exploring together a whole new world.

Every Aphasic Is Different

Our treasured feeling is that we are a very lucky pair.

Marvelous it is that there are thoughts and words and looks that do not have to be shared with anyone, and glorious is the path leading to the beauty of inviolate privacy.

As an aphasic I can't always explain how I feel simply by talking, for sometimes everything gets too involved for my mind to send directives to my brain, which must then give orders for speech. When that happens, my mate is alerted to my needs and wants by looks and gestures — maybe double whammy pantomime or loving caresses.

With such minuscule energy, my life becomes one compromise after the other: should I write a letter or clean the stove; should I do invoices or mop the kitchen floor; should I read a new book or straighten the mess into organized clutter? If I'm alone it will be the first things. If my Hans is due home the ties of love will rivet my attention to the latter duties.

I seem to be under a compulsion to do certain things right away: pay the bills the minute they arrive; be absolutely up to date on invoices, orders, financial and business records; get ideas typed while they are mentally visible lest they vanish into an unconscious wherever else.

The farther one gets from an experience, the dimmer become its outlines. And so it has been necessary for me to write things as they occurred to me in order for the recollections of my stroke to be as I thought they were during the first few days and weeks as I groped to right a reality that sometimes seemed topsy-turvy. It is possible to dig out "facts" you never knew were there, but that takes quiet, tranquil, open-ended thinking — one of the merits in aloneness.

Grateful am I that the stroke waited to descend on me until my daily responsibilities as a mother had ended. There has been thankfulness that it happened to me instead of My Dear, for it is easier for me to adjust to things that happen to me than to my mate. One perfectly good, practical reason for that is there is no financial strain.

I feel sure that my right hand would show greater improvement had I wanted to spend as much time retraining it as I have on writing. I could have had it pick up countless buttons; play rousing games of toss-up-cans-and-slam-them-down; use both hands to type, a nervewracking procedure if I want to accomplish anything.

More and more tasks are being done by my right hand. At its snail's pace it can dial the telephone, use the adding machine, help with lots of chores demanding both hands, but there just isn't enough energy for me to do, with equal success, both physical therapy and speech — in this case, that is writing, infinitely more meaningful to me.

There are three ideas I'd like to contest. Perhaps they are old wives tales, cultural hand-me-downs, ancient medical theories, but whatever they are they do not fit me.

1. A stroke means utter, absolute personal havoc.
2. Life is a desperate, back-breaking, heart-rending trial.
3. An aphasic is a temperamental wreck, bespeaking mountainous problems and God help the mate.

The stroke has not brought complete devastation to me. A stroke can be dreadful at best and aphasia unspeakable in more ways than one, but a stroke does not always completely wreck a life.

There are misconceptions. I have been told that I represent a miracle. I have also been told that my uneventful, "complete" recovery is natural since the stroke was so slight. But who really thinks about me: my reactions to aphasia, my background, my world of values, my approach to life, my marriage, what damage was done in my brain, my goals, my abilities, education, training, or even whether I have any sense?

If we have a glimmer of intelligence we know that no two people are exactly alike. Aphasics are people, and no matter what the *book* says they have reactions peculiarly their own. Perhaps part of the reason that aphasia is a paradox is because all its victims *are* different.

A point of philosophy that I find a bit nuts is the belief held by unbelievably many that life is a desperate, back-breaking, heart-rending trial from the pushing and shoving of birth through the agonies of death. Renegade that I am, life has not been so everlastingly hard for me, and its pricks and pains and jolts, together with its delights and joys, have led to greater understanding, more empathy with the world, as I see it.

Granted there are many, too many, people who have every reason to think life is a very bad trick to have played on them. And yet, often those who have the most complaints to make exhibit a poignant, spiritual awareness, a healthy, shining attitude.

And then let's look at this bit about aphasics and their personalities. Aphasia does a lot of dumb things but it really doesn't change the victim's basic traits. If one is happy, even-tempered and optimistic he is not apt to be a temperamental horror after aphasia.

We tend to interpret what others have written in the light of our own experiences and feeling and emotions and those do not always match the authors'. Be that as it may, there really are couples' like us who have successful marriages, who like being together, who enjoy meeting challenges, and who don't have problems even with aphasia.

And I say Hallelujah! Life wrapped in love is precious indeed.

7

The Nemesis of Fatigue

The Nature of Fatigue

It is startling to learn how few are aware of what a rapscallion fatigue can be — for many aphasics their consummate Nemesis.

Never have I known such overwhelming, sudden, inexplicable, complete fatigue — weariness so total that breathing becomes a chore. Now, when even taking a breath seems too much of a task how can one cope with anything?

Think what such devastating tiredness means to an aphasic: how does one explain that rest is needed — quiet away from every turmoil — when to say anything requires strenuous mental activity. It is incredible how few believe that. Take it from one who was probably born chattering, that is true — not just for the time the patient is hospitalized but maybe for the rest of his life.

Fatigue can be a demoralizing condition. There seem many logical reasons for being beset with tiredness and, yet, one of the characteristics of this sort of fatigue is that it may arrive without any apparent notice. One of its most endearing qualities is that it often descends with an almost audible kerplunk right after a surge of energy has zoomed through me. Then it is so unexpected I haven't time to find it either maddening or upsetting or even pokeable with a fork of humor. For me, it is easier to float with it rather than sink to a smothering depth for this kind of fatigue is a cousin to drowning.

It is said that aphasics are self-centered. At one time or another isn't everyone? Frustrated as an aphasic is by so many things ordinarily not even thought about, it is amazing he can think of anything or anyone while trying to get himself on an even keel. Do not be deceived: an aphasic's return to a "normal" life is precarious — having a little of the ham in him helps. Fatigue may be his constant shadow. Surely one does not have to be an aphasic to understand the totality of fatigue's impact.

A stroke rarely changes the patient's basic personality: if his milieu is his interest in others, that will continue to be his concern; if he is apt to moan and groan when things do not go as he wishes, then he may be highly resentful that such an outrage should have befallen him; if his attitude toward life is optimistic, he is likely to meet this peculiar disorder head-on.

When an individual has been clubbed by a stroke and aphasia it means there will, of necessity, have to be adjustments, so that others besides the patient may have an upset routine and some people can't stand to have their lives changed in any way. They may complain, "Why should we be the ones to make the adjustments?"

As for depression! Doctors and nurses are no exception — they, along with others, may THINK the patient is depressed because aphasia depresses THEM. The patient may be quite aware of this and becomes increasingly frustrated since he is unable to communicate.

Indescribable frustration may be felt by the aphasic, but one has to realize that those caring for him can be frustrated too. If everyone will remember that each aphasic is different, that aphasia hasn't really changed him, then patience alone will help to unlock a few doors. No one will deny that aphasia means adjustments, even gross ones, on the part of the patient, his family and/or others. If those involved can think of this blow as a challenge to the best in them and use imagination and perception accordingly, then this intelligent tackling of the inherent problems will have some good results. When aphasia is approached as a depressing disaster, one finds this kind of gloomy philosophy redounding to the patient and the results are not good.

The aphasic needs to learn to live contentedly with himself. He must not be subjected to coping with the discouragement of those around him, for though fatigue seems inevitable it need not be catastrophic.

This, truly, is the story of a fortunate aphasic: having the stroke when family responsibilities were on the wane; being sent to a hospital with a stroke unit; having a wonderfully understanding husband and family; the miracle of my speech therapist. What they all led to was a happy recovery and a successful rehabilitation — not complete but successful — and I'm still conked by fatigue.

Let's retrace our steps and see what was happening way back at the beginning. It was just a few days after the stroke up-ended me that I was able to take obnoxious sponge baths by myself and learned to get dressed with little or no help. Following these activities weariness assailed me, but by then it was time for breakfast. I was told that I was expected to do everything that might need to be done in the area of dining. That was fine and the thought that prompted this gentle kind of pushing was appreciated, but did any of the staff suspect what unmanageable fatigue I was experiencing too early in the morning?

My rescuer was my own good husband who was often there when most needed. He'd come bouncing in and when breakfast arrived he would shut the door, quite able to manage any displeasure his behavior might elicit. He did the necessary things — little things such as taking the top off the creamer and opening packets of sugar. Simple? Yes, and sometimes well nigh impossible. He succeeded in getting more food in me than could have been done on my own. He pampered me and I thrived and it was good.

Fatigue needs to be recognized by everyone who has anything to do with an aphasic for its import: it may play the leading role in an aphasic's life. People know that fatigue attends most aphasics, but few realize how total may be the aphasic's immersion in fatigue. It has been my experience that nothing can be done for very long at a time no matter how much the activity is a liked one, nor can "very long" be defined in terms of minutes for one's attention span is different at different times. At first, though, all sorts of things quickly became too much and still I couldn't tell anyone. (The perceptive speech therapist always knew. How her patients love her!)

Situational Experiences with Fatigue

Perhaps these two examples will give you an idea of apparently innocent experiences that seemed designed to produce zapping fatigue. The first one was while still hospitalized and the second one nearly two years post stroke.

Number One Experience – in the Hospital

Once on a happy time, three student nurses appeared in my room before I had quite awakened, and told me they were to be with me for much of several days. Oh Great Fish Hooks! Whose insane idea was that! They supervised my going to the bathroom, taking one of those hateful sponge baths, getting dressed, having breakfast, and if they weren't asking me questions they were whispering, mostly the latter, and taking notes – those must have been gloriously enlightening.

Then, they had to leave me – oh, just for a minute. They probably went unsupervised to a bathroom. They returned and took me in a wheel chair to the X-ray department which seemed to be way down in a sub-basement. There they were to be instructed in the kinds of X-rays which were to be used with me.

It seemed to take forever and afterwards they took me back, still whispering. As the patient, I couldn't help wondering what they were whispering about so much. I thought how much fun I could have if only I could talk and if I weren't so terribly weary. How could anyone be so tired!

Finally we returned to my room and they left me – alone – to have a nap, when in walked the physical therapist; and with that stint behind me, in came a nurse to take me back to X-ray. Woe is me! What happened to the first ones? If anyone knows no one is telling or it is classified information. Down we went minus my guardians.

Ultimately, the X-rays were finished and so was I, almost. The technician wheeled me into a waiting room of sorts and told me my floor had been notified. Opposite me was a receptionist, a clock and a mirror in which an apparition of a witch constantly appeared. And the minutes became nearly an hour. Finally the receptionist responded to my difficult-to-understand plea and in a few minutes a nurse arrived to take me to my room.

We had no sooner reached my sanctuary than Someone came in and the nurse explained to Someone how very tiring the morning had been for me but Someone snapped at me, "Now how could sitting make you tired?" If facial expressions are reflections of one's thoughts, why didn't Someone say, "What the hell does one do with this aphasic!" Bless that nurse! Because she knew and cared and had compassion she said, under her breath, but I could hear, — "Will That Someone never learn?"

Despite her uplifting, exhaustion precluded my eating lunch. I was even too tired for speech therapy which means my poor bashed brain was barely functioning. The therapist decided the morning had been entirely too much after one look at me, and especially after being haltingly told what it had been like — she is remarkable at understanding all when she gets almost nothing. Suffice it to say, my jail guards did not appear again and bless the one who saw to that.

It had been a morning full of lots of people, confusion, going and coming, understanding and misunderstanding perhaps not too different from an ordinary morning in a normal person's life. For me, even using my debonair manner reserved for sticky situations, it was an agony of weariness. Still, there were funny things about it: the ridiculous retorts that my mind gave me and which my brain rejected; that witch who kept a wary eye on me — enough to make me wonder what coven would accept her; the ingenious plans made for those cute student nurses to practice on themselves — dominant hand tied uselessly and no talking with ME supervising THEM.

And then to nudge my ego up a notch were the words of that perceptive nurse to whom my needs were more important at that moment than were hers or Someone's, and the intuitive wisdom and intelligence of the speech therapist. These were balances to help me view fatigue in proper perspective — it was dreadful fatigue but it did not become destructive. On that day, two dear, alert, wise women gave me the necessary sustenance to cope somehow with the tiredness.

Tiredness can be implacable, perhaps for every aphasic — certainly for me — implacable because it is forever lurking. When aphasia clouted me nature brought a mantle of insouciance which covered every usual sort of qualm but allowed my curiosity to run free. As awareness of what had happened really dawned on me, the enormity of it never once fazed me. The physical problems were dismissed with a mental shrug. Aphasia to me was a fuzziness in my thinking — an absolutely intolerable condition — and rightly so since, for as long as remembering, my one asset had been my mind. Yet there was no panic. The speech therapist would help me and studying was my forte.

Looking back at my work books brings a realization of the tremendous mental activity they represent. The fatigue, as it was, is certainly understandable but almost two years later to find it the governing influence in my life — what of that? That is understandable, too. Many, many simple, easy, every day functions cannot be done without conscious thought. For instance, speaking, incredibly easy once long ago, is now a puzzle to be solved. There are wonderful words gallivanting around my mind, but the right ones must be selected to see if they will fit the proper slot in my clunky brain and come out as requested. Maybe yes — maybe no — and maybe try again. Words will emerge only if spoken slowly — speech in slow-motion, and too much talking makes it ever harder to push out each word. Speaking *was* effortless — the marvel is that it can now be done at all.

But speaking is only one reason for fatigue. This next experience occurred nearly two years after the stroke and shows how an aphasic can be bombarded with events — each happening manageable but all of them mushrooming in geometric progression. The result: overwhelming weariness.

Number two experience — two years post-stroke

To maintain an inner equilibrium, I need to manage myself on my terms, a privilege my immediate family gives me. This second experience occurred while we were on a trip and for two nights there had been a brief approximation of the necessary sleep. On this particular morning, unknown to anyone but me, there were many signals that my faithful, if unwanted, shadow of fatigue was about to do his kerplunking landing. A late breakfast was eaten, reluctantly, but happily in the midst of those we love. Returning to bed was not feasible due to a meeting early that afternoon — one to which we were both looking forward.

Still silent about my tired insides, off we sallied. Our business was accomplished with such satisfaction that as we started for our home away from home that deceptive exhilaration swooped through me and then, suddenly, His Nibs said, "The adrenalin is gone. You need a nap."

Now our private traveling quarters are on wheels; we were

parked in a driveway and when we returned the fatigue was so great that just getting to bed was a monumental task. The danger point had been reached: sleep considered my pleas nonsense. The warning signals were sending SOS's chiefly to my tummy. This was a drowning tiredness. This was weariness when one dare not think, "Why aren't we home?" or "How are we ever going to do all we hope to do?" This was the kind of fatigue when one cannot think of the evening ahead — even of the next hour — only minute by minute by minute — floating with it — not whirling into its dizzying vortex . . . . The minutes grew into an hour — two hours — the tummy sensations subsided. Maybe the evening could be tackled, despite knowing what it portended: too many people however dear — too much noise — a beginning headache to be ignored. This was a situation in which an aphasic has to meet obligations — but to whom?

It may be difficult to explain why such a pleasant evening with good company, the murmur of nostalgic conversations, the laughter of rememberings, the lazy curls of smoke, the fine dinner, the fun afterwards should be recalled as havoc for me, Before dinner was over, a request was made for me to read my tribute to one not there in person and the request was refused. Did I care if someone else read it? Yes, I cared. I cared very much. It was the sort of writing to be savored alone and everyone there had read it. To tell them I cared, I nodded, or did I? Therefore, it was read by someone else and I retired to another room, not in a pique but because it was impossible to stay and listen. Could the wrong signal have been sent by me? If so, it was an aphasic flub.

Fatigue and unabashed sentiment, as companions, do not often lead to dignified reserve — rather, coupled, they are apt to provoke unsolicited tears. Oh, tears are not to be ashamed of, but they are difficult to handle when foreign to one's modus operandi. Difficult, too, for almost never are they understood. But my tears were not the only ones . . . . . . and the evening's festivities continued — more people arrived — old pictures were passed to and fro — reminiscences were gleefully told as memories unfolded — and finally, close to midnight. bed claimed me.

The entire next day was spent resting. This tiredness was so depleting that one day's rest was merely a start toward recovery and, as usually happens when fatigue becomes too great before a halt is called, the demon referred to as a headache was a calamitous though temporary intruder. By that night we decided maybe the dinner could be managed, and we tried. It went smoothly for me until a ridiculous argument began to be tossed from one wall to the other. Arguing with its pricks of venom has always been troublesome for me to listen to gracefully (now it's intolerable), and my perpetual role as a buffer is plumb kaput. My left hand came up and "stop" was spoken, neither of which brought one iota of relief. A firecracker exploded within me. . . . . I left the table, went outside to our mobile motel room and retired. This was more than I could cope with — much more. This was devastating fatigue.

Causes of Fatigue

You may ask, "Must an aphasic always be pursued by fatigue?" Perhaps no one has all the answers. This I do know: it cannot be a simple sleight of hand manoeuver for an energetic, enthusiastic, busy person to find his world in slow-motion — to find himself frustrated in areas he never dreamed possible. He needs every bit of discipline at his command to make adjustments, all kinds of them, and every day. If fatigue insists on trotting along with him, let him use it as a barometer to tell him how much he dare do and when he'd better stop. He needs — oh, how he needs — a rollicking sense of humor.

Fatigue is scarcely a condition belonging exclusively to aphasics, but it does seem that any factor causing fatigue is apt to be exaggerated in its impact upon an aphasic. Since we are all different, it isn't hard to understand that different things are important to us for different reasons, and so it is with fatigue. Each aphasic has his own lists of irritants capable of producing all-encompassing tiredness and probably no one list will be like any other.

For me, there are varying kinds of fatigue. My writing, which is my salvation, certainly produces weariness and yet it is a pleasant sort of being tired, especially after a session when words fairly tumble through the fingers of my left hand to become another typed page.

Attending to business details can be tiring, too, but there is satisfaction in being able to manage them for my Alter Ego, so it becomes a question of will this secretary-of-sorts know when to stop. Housework, anyone knowing me might think, should be at the head of the list of major irritants, but, since I have help and never was an impeccable housekeeper, the annoyance is likened to an occasional gadfly.

It seems to me that those things which cause the most frustration produce the most fatigue. With me those are:

> The inability to do more than one thing at a time
> Talking
> Social Affairs
> People
> Noise
> Decisions
> Driving
> Telephone
> Numbers
> Kitchen Scullery and Chores
> Pain

It is difficult to separate these categories completely — each seems to have at least one companion among some of the others and it is almost impossible to examine each one logically without having another one join the discussion. Therefore, if the following briefs seem like utter mish mash you will have to remember that decisions are a real bête noire for me. Perhaps it is not the effect of one factor of fatigue as much as their composite battering which so efficiently creates exhaustion.

Do one thing at a time

The inability to do more than one thing at a time is maddening. I was accustomed to juggling many activities at once: subtly watching teen children though supposedly paying no attention to them; doing invoices; discussing an issue needing immediate answers via the phone; jotting down ideas for a paper; and in and among these things successfully baking cookies the way this particular tribe likes them. It now seems unbelievable to find myself relegated to ONE activity at a time — ONLY ONE.

If it's exercising, then I must count. Wandering to a pleasant place in my thoughts and suddenly the counting sounds thusly: 7, 29, 50, 42, 68, 100 — interesting but hardly a rule of counting.

Walking with me is stimulating if one is expecting brilliant repartee. Ouch! My demented leg is not too noticeable but the fact is that it must be told, consciously told, where to go. With stairs to be manipulated, it must be told that there are steps to be negotiated or it will drag. If there is a branch or wire in the way that wacky kid bangs into it or stumbles over it unless told what to do.

My right hand and arm are amenable — not told what to do, they will do nothing. When told, the task will be accomplished, but not at my rate. Some satanic imp seems to have charge and annoys me by being incredibly slow and not always on target. Funny how that boob hand wobbles around in space trying to locate what it was told to find. Well, I didn't say rehabilitation was complete.

There have been those who have suggested in a rather peremptory way that both hands should be used in typing. It can be done, but it is easy to lose the thought on the detoured route of repairs through my brain to the paper especially when the right hand must be instructed about each letter to strike. Yes, it can be done. Is it worth what it does to me? It is frustrating, to put it mildly, and after a session of practice every muscle feels kinked. Rightly or wrongly, using only the left hand for typing prevents unneeded fatigue. You see, my mind flies fast as anything in many directions simultaneously, but it is unable to project thoughts or instructions through my clogged brain without untold mental effort.

Talking

Talking is wearing for me. Everything has to be thought of before speaking is attempted and even then it often emerges a trifle mixed up — *rand lover* for *land rover, spoking* for *soaking, value* for *valid, musician* for *museum, deaf* for *death, peepers* for *people* — these boo-boos are endless. Those don't bother me — sloppy speaking by me does: *hadda* for *have to* and *thass* for *that's.* The first kind of error is funny but the second sort is grating.

Talking is often one correction after another and there are times when tiredness blankets me so that I give up correcting even though aware of the errors — those are times when talking had better cease. Many have been the occasions when I wanted very much to tell someone something, but fatigue made it impossible. Paradoxical to have good thoughts, funny thoughts, helpful thoughts, nonsensical thoughts and no way to release them.

One professional person told me that he always has to think

before he talks and he didn't see why that should make it difficult to speak. That may be true for him. I only know that, prior to aphasia, I did not consciously think about every single phrase uttered by me — perhaps it would have been better if I had. Talking IS tiring but had I not worked so hard would it be as available as it is now?

Social affairs

A social affair! Once delightful — now a delirious confusion. If an outing involves more than six people it is apt to become one big mixture of noise. I cannot sort out conversations and if anyone asks me a question expecting an answer my voice won't generate enough volume so it becomes something which must be repeated or forgotten. Often there are refreshments to be reckoned with — a problem poser: how does one manage a plate of lovely snacks and a tall drink with a left hand and a lap — the right hand being so undependable that anything it clutches may be unceremoniously dumped all over the one next to me.

Now if anyone spots this creature without anything to eat — nothing to drink — in a twinkling sixty-'leven different souls are bringing me edibles and potables — still no place to put them so they hand them to me and rush off thankful that they have been so kind. After balancing them for a seeming eternity Mein Mann rescues me even as he mutters imprecations. Doesn't this sound relaxing?

If walking is necessary in a strange place, my dumb leg must know what to do, so a look-around advises what must be stepped over or up or down, my arm (the lazy one) must be told what to carry, no talking is possible — even were I to slip nothing will come, a proven fact — so it becomes a situation that is rather unworkable. The social affair is constant noisy confusion turning into a cacophony of sound and zap! awful fatigue.

Dining out can be a treat provided we are seated in a corner — at least some place where we are not surrounded by noisy people. If there is music, this seems to hit every spot in the room, resound, and track through me on its return trip. Since only one thing can be done at a time, eating and carrying on an intelligent conversation is not always easy. The added inconvenience — namely, that my swallower is not aware, sometimes, of signals telling it to work, or maybe the signals are late in arriving — whatever, this may find me with a mouthful of food, a question to be answered, and there I sit just waiting for another slow part of me to work. That is not catastrophic but it is wearing.

Another tiring factor is that usually the socializing and the dining out is at night and night finds me less than alert what with the zombies taking over my head. Anything may be said, words mangled, poor things, sentences completely dangling, and participles be danged. One redeeming feature is that our children find it amusing and have been known to say, "Mother, you're so funny. Say it again."

People

People! They can mean weariness which seems odd considering how important they have always been to me. Methinks one reason is that I'm a very private person — not everyone is a quite as private as myself needs to be. Most of my life there has been a spot to call my own, where everyone could be shut out and anything needing to be pursued could be, sustenance was found from my direct pipeline to Intelligence, and emerging from this place found me renewed. Maybe clean is the word, for there was a time when the only spot available was the bathtub.

Once upon a time the church on quiet week-days proved to be a marvelous retreat until snoopy ones got curious and ended what were truly moments of real refreshment. I love a church, only it is best if it's mine alone. Now if I'm considered a kook since being felled by a stroke, one can see that kookiness is a life-long quality.

A month in the hospital. It is doubtful if I could have stood easily anything less than a private room. Company was nixed and if the doctor had not insisted my husband would have. The door was to be shut most of the time — oh, this was NOT the doctor's idea — it was MINE and my mate was probably the only one who understood that.

To many of the personnel a shut door seemed to be equated with fear of facing anyone, although my attitude should have told them another story. I was not cantankerous. I didn't throw things, which doesn't mean that the thought hadn't romped through my mind more than once. The nurses were sweet and gracious about acceding to my wish that the door be closed but from other personnel there were almost daily lectures on the merits of an open door policy — these lectures were a source of irritation and fatigue. It seemed to me that my reasons were valid and anyone who thought otherwise was being obtuse. But, how could they know? I couldn't tell them.

While still hospitalized it was suggested that I plan to have tea parties for the neighborhood when enthroned at home — a suggestion that sent cold chills clear through me. Tea Parties! Those are marvelous for the very young in their first experiences with Winnie-Ther-Pooh and Kanga but now? Why do I need to be surrounded by people and ones I am supposed to entertain at that? That means getting the house in order, preparing something to eat — a completely exhausting idea and one dismissed vehemently and as fast as possible.

My friends have been wonderfully understanding. They have known — because they know me — if recovery was to be successful it was going to have to be on my terms. Visiting was done when they carted me to therapies for three months. They knew business details would be tackled by me at home. They hoped I would write. They have not overwhelmed me with visits. They have been generous with notes — cautious about calling. They are loved ever more. There have not been tea parties!

Thinking about crowds of people is fatiguing in itself. I avoid shopping — never one of my delights — even grocery shopping is not easy. If by myself, I get as few things as possible, go when fairly sure there will not be hordes, send someone else when feasible, and thus it is a matter of subtly by-passing unwanted and unneeded fatigue.

Where most any number of people were manageable, now confusion reigns unorganized if I am surrounded by them. When my role is to answer questions while sitting before people telling them what aphasia has been like for me, then I am not bothered no matter how few or how many people there are, for that is a controlled situation. Nor does it disturb me to make mistakes or have difficulty finding the right word.

Each aphasic needs to decide what he can do and what he wants to do and then whack out all the extraneous stuff he can live comfortably without doing. Despite the element of fatigue, it is important to me that interested people see and hear me and, it is to be hoped, gain a little more insight into what it can mean to one to be an aphasic. Writing my thoughts about this baffling disorder may be another bridge of enlightenment between some aphasic and those around him. Discouragement, a tremendously tiring attitude, could be rife on both sides. It does not need to be.

Noise

Noise is a factor in fatigue that cannot be overlooked. There was a day, long before aphasia came to be with me, when I came home from our office to find my helper surrounded with noise of all kinds — amazed that she could tolerate the racket the children were imposing upon her. In the room where she was ironing, a ping-pong game was being played, the t.v. was on loud as could be, the radio was giving forth unbearable yowls called music, from the area of the sprouts' bedrooms a record player was blaring with equally unbearable screeches, and in the midst of this the telephone jangled and conversation was carried on. How? Who knows! If you find yourself encircled with children of varying ages you will recognize this as a loud but not really an abnormal situation. Now if, at this point, I found myself in the middle of such a raucous ruckus would it be bearable? The answer is a definite NO! What of the aphasic who must live with this commotion, with any kind of a situation equally hard for him to manage without dreadful fatigue?

It would be salutary if everyone intimately involved with an aphasic could know for one whole day the fatigue that stalks many aphasics constantly. Attitudes might be changed full circle and fatigue-producing factors such as noise would be muted if not eliminated. It is a happy thought but is it only a dream?

While still in the hospital, any noise bothered me and, although there probably was not too much, anyone who has spent time in one knows that in the area of quiet a hospital leaves much to be desired. What better reason could there have been for wanting the door closed? I needed to concentrate on speech therapy assignments and any distraction made the laborious task of forcing an idea through my caved-in brain to the paper even more tedious and tiring.

Noise still has a deleterious effect on me. A week-end of ball games leaves me internally agitated, externally more aphasic than usual; it becomes harder to think straight — takes longer to decide anything — the Monday following such bombarding two days is likely to be a very tired day. That is a day when it seems virtually impossible to do much. Typing thoughts, which is a pleasure, leaves me with an empty feeling because on that day nothing will come right. The thoughts are there, but it is the wrong time for translating ideas into words that make sense. There have been occasions when an entire day is spent writing a paragraph deemed unusable by me. That truly is a tired day.

The peacefulness of the house all to myself is the most renewing sort of aloneness — not the absence of noise but the quality of sound. Noise, if allowed to go beyond the limits an aphasic can endure, becomes brutal in its inward attack. Lovely sounds heal a bruised spirit: the wind playing tag with the squirrels on the roof top; the birds gossiping to each other; the house audibly creaking as it settles for a nap; the fire crackling on the hearth; raindrops tapping lightly on the panes — all of them nature's heart's-ease and comfits.

Perhaps the sorts of noisy clamors that bother me have been the same clangings that have always been a nuisance — only now they have a more exaggerated impact on my innards. They become the kinds of things one must accept as factors to be avoided if gracious equilibrium is to be maintained.

Decisions

Decisions! Oh, but this is a fun part of my aphasia! And they had never been difficult for me prior to being bashed by this weirdo. There was never any doubt about the first decision which actually I was not permitted to make. It was completely unimportant to me that part of me refused to work at all. With my thinking so foggy, who could feel that *anything* took precedence over getting my thinker percolating again.

It is my assessment that the patient has the right to decide where he wants to give most of his extremely limited energy: physical therapy or speech. It will not be the same for every patient. My impression is that not one whit of attention was paid to my distinct preference for speech except by the speech therapist.

As for current decision problems, they are decisions about everyday things: what will be worn; what shall we have for dinner; what do we need from the grocery; will this house ever look like anything more than a city dump; and how much of this ucky junk can be disposed of — things about which almost all feminine creatures have to decide. True, but almost all femmes aren't aphasics. It's just that a lot of the special ones who are aphasics find it harassing to deal with such picayune problems.

One perplexing dilemma for me is found in the adventure called dining out. There is an item on the menu which sounds tempting and it is ordered for me. Fine. . . . . Presently the waitress comes with the news that the restaurant is out of my choice, something else must be selected. Agony! It does seem as though it would be easier if foods were my forte. Hopefully, my spouse will help depending on the state of my speechlessness. Then appears the waitress and her list of appetizers: we have turtle soup, tomato juice, pigeon eggs wrapped in bacon, fruit cup ambrosia, or squashed chicken livers. I'll probably say "vichyssoise, please." This goes on with vegetables, salad dressings, and oh yes — drinks: coffee, tea, limeade, lemonade, milk, or beer. Hot tea, please. No hot tea but we have iced tea. I'll have a frozen daiquiri. Spell that fatigue in capitals! After several sessions with these unnerving decisions, the solution is to let my partner in marriage, children and business do the ordering.

Another decision kind of nonsense is having to tell workmen in the house or the yard or the street or on the roof EXACTLY what to do. That is a NO — a double-deckered, triple lettered N-O-O!

Lady Luck has smiled on me bountifully since my sparring with aphasia. The super helper we had had for over two decades, unavoidably elsewhere, was able to return to us one day a week, and by the time she was free she arrived with a shovel, a pick-ax, a hose, and three gallons of Chlorox.

Calling our home a disaster area is entirely too mild an opprobrium. It does not seem possible that the many minute instructions could be given by me to anyone who had not helped us, and why? That is more than I could cope with at this point.

Our sterling gem knows where everything is, she knows what to do and does not need to be told anything. She is perceptive and understanding and has been a part of this family for such a long time. There is no energy for me to enlighten anyone on where equipment is, what must be done, how, etc. etc., ad nauseam. An unfamiliar someone in the house all day? No! My dear helper is used to the odd things I do — like talking to myself. No doubt someone unknowing would think me crazy especially when she couldn't understand me.

Truth is: it's easier to have a crummy house than go through the misery of breaking in help. That kind of fatigue is not needed. Right now it is an item requiring no thought, and perhaps if it ever does I will feel differently. It may be a matter of having a soupçon more energy and feeling more confident in my abilities to wrestle with run-of-the-mill problems — for instance, housework. Once it meant travel to shining places or figuring out pat solutions to perplexing human puzzles and presto! the housecleaning was done, but alas, aphasia has quashed such delightful freedom and sentences me to one activity at a time.

What is it about decisions that makes them so wearing? For that matter, what are decisions? Don't they mean assessing one idea, then another, perhaps several others, then putting all the components together, readjusting and making judgments. It does seem to me, no matter how unscientific this may be, that thoughts must be programmed through one's brain. Since the stroke has exterminated some of those neat little slots, new ones must be found; and when an aphasic has a decision to make, he may find himself in totally unfamiliar territory. By the time he locates a different route he may have forgotten why he needed it. The meadow of one's mind may be fairly serene, but the danger lies in those inevitable trips through the brain to the world outside — deliberate and labored treks.

The enormity of what aphasia can mean is appalling even with only a glimmer of understanding, and where is it more exacting in the fatigue it causes than in the area of decisions? With me decisions seem to be hardest in those areas where there is the least interest and easiest in areas having the greatest interest. The considered thought once expended on decisions now seems automatic compared to the amount of effort they extract from me today.

Driving

Driving! For the nonce there are many reservations, all mine, about my abilities as a driver, although even my husband, with his high standards, considered me a good one.

At the suggestion, encouragement, and pushing of those expected to know about aphasics, I have driven since the eighth month post-stroke. Under ideal conditions, the time from home to office should be twenty minutes. Can you imagine what it must be like taking all the back lanes (lanes sound easier), going by lights only, letting cars pass if it means pulling to the curb, and arriving at the destination feeling like an unravelable knot. Are you a bit woozy just hearing about it?

The ego-boosting driving gives to many — the wonderful feeling of independence — is not worth the kind of fatigue driving imposes on me. And so it seems better to go only to places easy to get to, at times when fewer cars will be on the road and children in school safe from me. My before-stroke nightmare is worse then ever: that a child will suddenly appear. Will my reaction be correct?

Funny how my confidence returns once driving is under way. Using a twirling knob the driving is handled easily as a southpaw. When asked, "Why don't you use both hands?" the answer is that my right hand is willing — too willing — clamps the wheel violently, and refuses to let go.

Returning home from an excursion in the car finds me with

a triumphant, exhilarated feeling that everything was fine, a few threatening situations managed with aplomb, no reason not to tackle any driving. BUT, then comes the realization that muscles are squinched up tight and fatigue doesn't settle gently over me — it clobbers me. Then I'm not so sure that driving is easy. Oh, perhaps it will be done, but only the simple places, remembering that even those spots can sometimes be hazardous.

Telephone

And then there's the telephone which can be monstrous — at least to this aphasic. Is it the numbers which can easily be reversed or the fact that the person called or calling can't be seen or is there uneasiness that I will forget to whom I am speaking or what was called about? It must be remembered that never has telephoning been one of my acute pleasures.

Calls from friends are gratefully received; telephone selling is abhorred; business calls are accepted reluctantly and made the same way. One of the first business calls made by me was a darb! The phone rang several times before being answered and by then the name of the firm "had fallen out of my mind." In my inimitable fashion, the one who answered was given my name and told, frankly, that the reason for calling had been misplaced somewhere in my bing-banged brain. Judging by the interminable length of time it took me to tell her this, she knew something had to be a bit wrong and bless her — whoever she is, bless her *mille fois* — she directed exactly the sorts of questions needed to dig out the misplaced information, and she manipulated the episode with real concern and sweet talk, making the whole affair one to be remembered thankfully and not with the distaste of failure.

It was fine to have this so-right person handle this stage-struck aphasic, insecure in my ability to manage the telephone. She has helped me more than she could possibly have known. There have been a few near-failures, but always could be heard that sweet concerned voice — in effect, a memory steadying sound — and somehow my desires were made known and the calls turned out to be successes after all.

Almost any kind of phone call that can be made has been made by me, so the success that lies in achievement has been mine. Trying to see a task through to completion is often accompanied by needless worry when the actual doing becomes fairly routine. This is surely part of my difficulty with the telephone — if not all. It is strange that an instrument of communication can be so miraculous and such a monster. It can produce, for whatever reasons, very real, an almost palpable fatigue in me.

Numbers

Together, the telephone and numbers can be comically disastrous. There have been occasions when, during the course of the call, a number has been asked for, though not available, and then, while the call had been initiated by me, the one called was told quite saucily, it must be admitted, to forget the whole thing. And when the receiver was replaced, not too gently, I yelled, "I hate being a number!" followed by the only cuss words that would come, not too bad, worse were thought but refused to climb that delapidated trail to the outside world. Numbers can be so frustrating and so tiring!

My tongue gets twisted as well as my brain, and numbers are terribly hard to duplicate correctly over the phone. One favorite bookstore, where much delightful browsing has been done and most of our book business transacted, spoiled it all when one sad day a great big number was the only acceptable way business could be accomplished. No longer was I a person — a real, live human earth person. I was a number. We have changed bookstores and what will happen when or if this accomodating company also decides that customers are numbers? It will be a messed-up day for me.

In my business duties, numbers are found in a milieu where only simple arithmetic is required. One of my tasks is totaling invoices which must then be entered in the proper column. Then, there are daily figures of numerous kinds to be tabulated and market week figures; there are bank accounts to be balanced and provided periodically with enough money to cover the bills. I checked a bank statement one month post-stroke. It was right to the penny but oh, it took me such a long, long, wearying time. This kind of work must be exact and though fatigue may sneak up on me right after feeling exceptionally peppy, it is not the crunching kind frustration is wont to bring.

Numbers can make me very tired, and they become more difficult at night. Night is when Hans calls and, among other items to relay to him, there may be pull-outs in one of his lines which means reading their numbers. It is so easy to err: the number is 25913 or was it read as 39512? Sometimes I will say the wrong number out loud, but repeat the right one in my head — maybe it was wrong both places — blankety blah!

Numbers, the kind that show we are doing fine, are great. It is the kind one finds on charge plates that make me mad as an untranquilized orangutang. I'd rather be a letter. Think what could be done with x: xanthin − xenomia − xyst − xylophone. But numbers! They are so putridly, pusillanimously impersonal! Besides that, for me they are called fatigue.

Kitchen Scullery and Chores

Kitchen scullery is another tiring activity. Females, if they are sensible and at all proper, are supposed to be devoted to kitchens in a wholeheartedly domestic way − or is it that we are told that. Maybe my genes weren't assorted very well. Any way one looks at it, it is a supposition or superstition that doesn't fit me. Not that the kitchen is loathsome, but it inspires me only to do what has to be done as quickly as possible.

Since aphasia, it is even less inspiring and you know why? The same old reason: once kitchen stuff could be done with my mind gallivanting to blazingly amazing spots and then it was fun. But now, there is an imposed curse of do only one thing at a time!

There is one little deviation that has added scorching interest. My lazy hand, if not told what to do, does nothing except when near the oven and then, prodded by Satan or memory, it comes sneaking up for a look-see and a help-touch-burn. It's happened half a million times, enough to wear a body clear down to the nub. The nitty gritty of it is that I murmur a feeble no to most kitchen details.

Now there's another mixed-up pattern that has come since aphasia decided to live with me. It is noticeable particularly in the kitchen chores: my left hand is now my dominant hand and so it thinks it is the right hand. Invariably, one can find me trying to use my left for my right and my right for who knows what and the upshot of this peculiar activity is as though some jerky demon was afflicting me with the mumbo-jumbo hebejeebees. With these exasperating motions, edibles are brought slowly and carefully and one at a time to the table. How to keep hot foods hot and cold foods cold! What a tiring confounded mess!

Then, of course, there seems to be a goofy imp in charge of my taste buds. Rarely do things taste good − more often than not food tastes spoiled or like used motor oil or half-cooked cardboard. Do you wonder why the kitchen is boring?

Fatigue must surely have a lot to do with eating or should it be the other way around? My tummy seems to be the same one that has always belonged to me, but, sadly, it is cast-iron no longer and the current workable rule is to eat little at a time and eat more frequently. If certain signals come from my midriff it is time to call a halt to the activity engrossing me — no matter what it is. That's called foiling fatigue, but if not one bit of attention is paid to warning signs it strikes again: unremitting fatigue.

The things that have made me the most frustrated have been in those nuisance areas where we normally expect to use both hands — frustrating and tiring. My left hand has managed to do many things it was unaccustomed to doing but it needs training in an Atlas Physical Strengthening Program.

Minor details, such as taking the top off of toothpaste, unscrewing the lid on a jar of coffee, removing the top on preserves or pickles, opening pre-packaged anything, pose problems where there ought not be any. One occupational therapist told us about a one-handed can opener which is great and a special knife which works well.

Most difficulties of this nature involve such simple tasks — easily done if there are people to do them, but when the aphasic is alone they can be maddening and these irking nuisances will differ from one aphasic to another. When one has been used to doing things for himself, it is a strange sensation to find he is dependent on others in areas he never would have expected.

These are problems needing concerned thought, imagination and a whole big bunch of love. Little things are often the worst and the hardest for everyone involved. Simple, silly, top-lifting problems can develop into irritating, severe frustration. Still, somewhere there are solutions. They may appear at the most unlikely times and from the most unlikely sources but they will come — an aid to everyone's frustration and fatigue.

Pain

To my amazement, pain is a factor in fatigue difficult for me to manage. A recent session with bursitis and treatment, never a delight, was almost unbearable, and since the arm was my good one, there were unbelievable moments in this comedy of ouches.

You will be spared the more vivid details, but for several days my life was a bit cruddy — the only tolerably comfortable spot was in a tub of hot water and even then the top refused to budge on a marvelously fragrant bath oil which would have been balm for my soul. Maybe it would have fortified me for the torture of getting out — a manoeuver which very nearly undid me.

It was a week before I could do much of anything. If there is a next time — Heaven Forbid — maybe it should be while My Dear is home, though really he ought not to be subjected to the moans and groans and tears of pain and fatigue at its worst.

It took weeks for me to regain the energy lost in that encounter. Was it because I had so little reserve? Eating had to be indulged in every few ten minutes and it was easier to drink stuff like Jello and sweetened condensed milk — then back to bed to get enough energy to get up and eat or drink some more. It was plumb awful — like groping around in some dank, dark dungeon.

It doesn't make much difference what the reasons are, the fact remains that pain is a big factor in fatigue where it used to be lumped with all the other irritants and managed without too much ado. It always was a bother — now it seems to be an exaggerated symptom bringing with it unmanageable weariness.

Reactions to Fatigue

Tears

A reaction that is a part of fatigue with me, and perhaps with lots of aphasics, is tears. Normally, I shed very few — principally because a crying jag gives me a dreadful headache and that is a torment to avoid at any cost. A young lady, known to me, can cry and her blue/gray/touch-of-green eyes become a shining, exquisite aquamarine. To do that and not have a fiendish headache might afford me enjoyment and relief but, as it is, crying, if witnessed, is a torture — not even indulged in often when alone, since for me tears seem to have only detrimental effects. Even so, there sometimes are sudden, momentary tears for no apparent reason — probably there have been too many people, too much to cope with, too many misunderstandings, too many dumb thises and thats — voila! a few tears.

Yes, fatigue can be the source of many tears and yet, it seems that rarely are tears associated with an aphasic's fatigue — always they seem to spell depression. Nuts! True, depression must be fatiguing and true, depression and fatigue may produce tears, BUT tears do not have to mean the aphasic is depressed. They may signal frustration, anger, fear, gratitude, relief, sentiment, happiness, having one's emotional control center smashed. Or simply fatigue.

130

Depression

Depression has to be fatiguing. Conversely, fatigue could produce depression if one is exhausted, is prone to pessimism, and if he feels that no one understands what is happening including himself. It must be a ghastly pit to try to climb out of only to slip back again and again.

Maybe I don't know what depression means. One standard definition describes it as "a condition of general emotional dejection and withdrawal; a sadness greater and more prolonged than that warranted by any objective reason."

I have read that stroke patients are almost universally depressed. I can only discuss my own reaction. I am an aphasic. By the above definition I have never been depressed. I could have been had the stroke occurred even a year earlier, had circumstances been different. Oh, there may be any number of reasons why depression could have inundated me.

But I certainly have plumbed the depths of fatigue. To lead me through these trials by fatigue have been my two miraculous assets: an understanding, loving husband and a perceptive, wise speech therapist. I said I was a lucky aphasic and so I am.

The Balance-Wheel Philosophy

There really is no way to know all the untold alphas and omegas which go into making us as we are. What we know of ourselves may be only a small part of each of us as a total microcosm, but this I know about me: I have always had everything I ever wanted my whole life. The stroke has been considered a challenge and met head-on by me and my mate.

Fatigue is the signal everyone has that renewal time has come. It may come through sleep, change of pace, an interlude of sitting by the fire watching dreams, by whatever means each one finds his private source of feeling at peace with himself.

Many of us as aphasics find much more time is needed to gain even an elusive spurt of energy and our most effective renewing channels need to be sought more often if we are to present any real equilibrium to our world — probably a more circumspect world than it had been before aphasia. But that world is one in which we should feel free to try our banged-up wings, to do anything our hobbled selves will enable us to do, to pursue old hobbies and if those are now unworkable try new ones. It is possible to change the direction of a life.

Nothing is impossible for the spirit: it can soar over any mountain, feel its way through any jungle and when tired, glide happily down the wide river of thought. Truly a blessing, since most aphasics face a mountain of problems in communication and a jungle of misunderstandings. If every aphasic could have one person — one balance wheel — he would have less trouble learning to come to grips with himself and to manage a constant shadow, fatigue.

Two balance wheels have I. They create fun and interest in life as it is now, help me use such talents as are mine, and make it feasible for me to manage without disaster that eternal bug-a-boo called fatigue. These are the nudges everyone needs to grow in the dimension of the spirit; wonderful antidotes for fatigue and malaise are balance wheels, those infinite circles of perception, understanding, intelligence and love.

8

Bits And Pieces And Au Revoir

This brings me to two and one-third years beyond the morning when aphasia, with no discernible warning, came to stay with me. Occasionally, my head shakes "no" for "yes," an error I may or may not catch. Or a name is mentioned. Do I know it? Yes, but at that moment the reason how or why eludes me in favor of emptiness.

There are still funny aphasic spellings: *Milwaukee* turns out *Milkauwee; blame* emerges as *blaim; entirely* comes forth *enretily; been* and *seem* forever being spelled *benn* and *semm*. Sometimes one needs an interpreter to decide what I've written. Pronunciation is still problematical: *worse* for *worth; kite* for *quite;* slushing and sliding, with words forgetting they are separate bits and pieces of a puzzle not easily solved when they all mush together.

In this final chapter there will be thoughts on these topics:
1. From a time clock of 2-plus years things that are

bothersome to me;

2. Reaction of others to me as an aphasic;
3. The status of aphasia as seen by me and some philosophical implications.

Time-Clock: Two-Plus Years. Yield: Bothersome Things

To be in my own home provides me with ways — intellectual, emotional, spiritual — to make my life satisfying. Need anyone ask for more? A spot of comfort, a private, lovely retreat — my home has always meant that to me as busy as my life had been.

It was geared to people. It could be said they surrounded me. My life is still geared to people, but from a different vantage point. Whatever can be done by me to make aphasia more understandable will be done, and writing is a good way whether it is for many or for one. Talking and looking at people may put a double hurdle on the track, and often I find myself either shutting my eyes or looking off in space in order to persuade the right words, or any words, to leave their cozy nest in my mind to traverse the rocky road through my brain to the outside world.

Aphasia, in one sense, could be called a disorder of exaggeration: Too much of anything comes too soon. Too many people, too much noise, too many distractions, too much to see. Things that normally impinge on our visual and auditory senses can bring total fatigue quickly, an aspect of aphasia which is not easy to cope with and difficult for many to comprehend.

This exaggerating surfeits my life in quite a few places. For instance, there is shopping for groceries. Once it was fun, even a hurry-up trip, perhaps acquaintances to chat with on the run or wave to, but now unless planned carefully . . . . . ??!!

First, I must be sure to have a grocery list and plenty of money. Then a drive to the store with, hopefully, no encounters. Prior to the stroke, difficulty in driving was never thought of consciously. Now it nags so much that driving may mean setting a goal of one block at a time until reaching the destination. Driving demands being constantly alert every old which way and able to zip an instruction through a brain that is set on slow motion. But aphasia demands doing one thing at a time. Getting those two demands to mesh means driving is exhausting for me.

Finally, or so it seems, the super market is reached, the car parked, and a deep breath girds me for the next round. Since this is an excursion that has been put off for several days, the list of needed supplies is rather imposing and my way is wended up and down the aisles, but why is it so difficult to find the products on the list? Here are the crackers and looking for the two kinds wanted seems futile, so searching begins section by section, row by row and after an interminable (to me) length of time one kind is located and then the other.

This is not an unusual occurrence. It happens over and over, up and down most every aisle, for there are too many things to look at and the ones being hunted don't pop out visibly the way they did once upon an easier time. Standing is deadly, so the longer it takes to find products the more weariness pours through me and that means it takes even more time to locate the next item. If only there were a box to sit on for a refreshing moment . . . .

This combination of tiredness, frustration, wooziness may mean stopping STAT and getting only the groceries already piled in the cart. Has it ever occurred to me to walk out of the store empty handed? Indeed it has, but lectures to myself have made it possible to get through the check out counter and back to the car intact with a few groceries if not all that should have been purchased.

Then a few moments of recovery before tackling the final lap of getting home. Can you bring yourselves to imagine the consummate relief at finding myself in my own house once more safely if shakily, knowing there may be another better time but that is in the 'to-do' file and doesn't have to be thought about this relieved, safe moment.

Would not most of you refer to a stint of grocery shopping as a very ordinary doing? Yet, here is a "recovered" aphasic who finds it a challenge which often turns out to be a torture if not a near disaster. 'Tis an event which always has to be approached with renewed positives.

How should this iffy situation be handled? Let's take it bit by bit. Driving is the one area in which my confidence is kaput. It wasn't when driving began eight months post stroke, for although there was uneasiness there wasn't a complete lack of confidence. Now that driving has been a possible feat for a year and a half why this sudden feeling of impending disaster that refuses to be shaken?

There have been two experiences that could have been

accidents but were not. The first happened one day as I was moseying along a street minding my own business but quite aware of traffic, when suddenly right next to me a horn blared, reason unknown. Horn noise can be infuriating because it is usually unnecessary and the loud blast startled me sufficiently to make my arm jerk which sent my car up over the curb and back down again. No, nothing happened BUT there were cars in front of me, behind me and beside me, and nowhere to stop for a few moments while my innards were properly rearranged. It was frightening and that day there was real mental celebration when home was reached with car and me intact.

Two weeks after this incident the second occurred in a parking area where, normally at that hour, there wouldn't have been many cars. That day it was jammed. There was one empty space and I eased into it at the proper angle but, instead of braking as we came to a rolling stop, the accelerator was stomped . . . . Fortunately, the curb was high enough to prevent jumping it. How could I have done such a stupid thing that might have resulted in a terrible tragedy? A prayer and sheer nerve got me home. The only casualty was my confidence which is still lying where it flew out of me and the car and by now it's been so trampled retrieving it is doubtful.

The solution to that part of the grocery buying problem would seem to be to have someone else take me to the store, which is usually the way it is managed. The next step is to go at an hour when traffic is not heavy for that means there are fewer people to contend with, fewer carts to watch out for, fewer distractions. I am less rushed about telling my pokey right foot where to go, find hunting for items less hectic which means all of our needs will be located, and getting through the check out counter is apt to be a minimal problem.

In doing any sort of shopping, it is not the shopping proper that is bothersome but the extraneous components of people and noise. Those two factors, combined with the necessity of alerting my foot about the terrain being trod, make a major excursion out of any trip where buying is the intention. When any kind of shopping can be turned into a spectator sport, with me riding and sitting in the car watching people while others do the work, it solves lots of problems.

One interesting aspect of my aphasia is the difficulty in sorting things, be they cans of soup, books, furniture, words in a newspaper, cars or sounds. It can be a slam bang jumble of foreground and background.

It is found in trying to sort out voices and conversations, noticeable particularly at parties or in dining out where there are many people, so that the noise of talking is not a subdued humming but a raucous screeching making it impossible to understand anything directed at me. It is found in stores where every display is a plethora – a very big too muchness. How can anything be selected if one is overwhelmed by sights and sounds?

It is found in newspapers for they are too bulky, too much, too busy. It is found in driving or riding for there are too many cars, too close, too noisy. Noise, people, products equal too much too soon and so a foreground/background tangled mix-up. These auditory-visual distortions are still troublesome. Will they always be?

One can't resign from the human race just because he's been granted membership in the exclusive, select club of aphasia and I discipline myself into doing those things I would rather not do. There's always the happy thought that this will be the time when everything will go smoothly and I will be glad to have done whatever it is I ought to do. Every aphasic's list of don't-want-to-do will be different but this much is certain: whatever has happened to us, nothing will improve until we do something constructive about it ourselves.

You've heard about the frantic, frustrated, frazzled me. What about the rest? One of the nice things about being a marvelously fashioned human is that there are so many yous and mes. And that has advantages. Nobody likes to be frantic, frustrated, frazzled, that self being one we'd like to discard or deny or ignore only we won't if we have any sense. Maybe it can be sandwiched between the happy self and the contented self.

Who is the happy self? The one who enjoys visits from children and friends; who likes to see relatives and friends in their native habitats; who is eager for adventures alone with That Man; who is delighted to appear before any group at any time in the interests of aphasia.

And the contented self? One left at home alone; letters and ideas waiting to be pushed through my brain to be expressed via the typewriter; invoices to be sorted and tabulated; bills to be paid; books to be tasted; thoughts by the dipperful to be quaffed from the fountain of endless knowledge; nature's vibrant, changing scene to be enjoyed from a window; moments with My Dear to be cherished . . . . the purring me.

These are a few of the many mes as they are viewed by me, myself. How I appear to others I really am not sure, but I do know that reactions of people to me since I stumbled and fell into a stroke trap have been almost as varied as all of our selves put together.

There are those wonderful ones who always accept me the way I am; use their eyes and ears and heads to determine how things are, what can be done and what cannot; play their part accordingly and then reassess the situation when they see me the next time.

There are those to whom the word *stroke* seems to be so shocking that I, the victim, feel I am polluting the entire atmosphere. There are those who cannot bring themselves to use the word, though one is not sure whether by ignoring the subject of a stroke it and its effects will go away, or whether the person thinks the subject is too painful for me to discuss. So I use the word, at least stumble through it for it is a hard word for me to pronounce, and the listener seems to cringe.

There are those who show relief when they realize my marbles are where they ought to be. Some of them tell me, some squeeze me. But what if it were well nigh impossible to speak clearly; what if the intended words emerged as something totally different; what if some words said to me didn't make much sense; what would they think then? Verbal communication, speaking and interpreting, is so vital to being a human that many assume when one loses that ability one loses his mind. His mind is still churning, probably working overtime. It's his brain that's been bashed.

There have been those who have said, "Come on, you couldn't have had a stroke. You aren't a stroke-prone person." A bit of probing revealed their thinking that one was a candidate for a stroke if she were a tempestuous harridan. Now if they haven't seen much overt display of temper, maybe it's because mine is the kind that 'susplodes' internally and that much tension could cause some devilish disarrangements. *Voila! Peut-être c'est moi.*

Then it has been announced to me in no uncertain terms, "Yes, I might have known it. You're still a pollyanna." Would a sour puss, a weeping, complaining old hag be more acceptable? Or are some offended by pollyannas because they cannot possibly be happy themselves? Pleasing everyone is so impossible, it is surely best to concentrate on pleasing the nearest and dearest ones.

And the suggestions! They should have been collected like pretty pebbles in a jar. Sadly, most have gone in and out the sieve that is a stand-in for a brain, but this remembered one was graciously delivered with solemn authority: "Tell you what you should do. Get you an old fashioned iron, a real iron. Any good junk shop will have one. Carry that in your right hand wherever you go — and I mean everywhere — even if you get up and move to another chair, carry the iron with you. I guarantee it won't be any time before that hand is as good as it ever was. And that's all you have to do. Much better than any exercises."

We had comical visions of my fingers clutching the handle of an iron, glued to it so that they and it could never be separated. We didn't find a real iron. Truth is, we never looked. But a few days ago nail clippers were used by my right hand. With or without the iron, how's that for progress!

Philosophical Tid Bits

There are days when everything smiles on me as though this is a day anything can be done — a marvelous feeling even if it doesn't last for long. And there are days when the only reason for getting up is because of that turning-to-cement sensation in my joints which creak and crack as some of the stone work breaks off and so getting up is easier than miserably lying in bed.

Days when walking seems like weaving and even imaginary twigs are stumbled over. On these tottery days one wonders if a walking stick would help, but after falling over nothing the conclusion is reached that it would be another thing to watch. Days when ideas pour from mind to brain to typewriter and days when they slide like quick sand through my mind and refuse to stop their chase of each other long enough for me to capture one.

Days when doing anything requires more energy than can be mustered and days when the got-to-get-it-done self pushes beyond reasonable limits knowing full well what will happen, but able to look at that wretched happening squarely with a snide smug of 'it got done so there, smarty.' Comfortable days when everything seems to be going well for everyone. Fun days spent on our bluebonnet hill wondering what kind of a house we would like the best.

These are interesting days. Some would call them days retrieved from eternity. I do not feel it can be assumed that my life here is being operated on borrowed time, for time in its cosmic definition is eternal. But each day is precious, for in that brief span it is possible for us to seed ideas by words or actions which might eventually bring forth a veritable harvest of wonder. With all the ideas glimpsed, exciting, awing, constructive does there need to be destruction?

Has there ever been such a cliff hanging moment in our history as now? Will the marvels, the goodness surface or will our planet be submerged, like Atlantis, drowned by human catastrophes? Those of us to whom planting ideas may be the only constructive responsibility left to us better get busy and plant. The ultimate harvest will be exhilarating even if we aren't participating here.

In this age when it is possible to go to the moon and back; when a neuron can be dissected a to izzard; when new math is touted, although a bank statement won't balance unless a 4—4=0 not a +7 or a —5; when spare parts can be transplanted and what a day it will be when a brain — ? Don't hold your breath but give that one to your mind to chomp on for recreation; in this wonderful age of inventions, abilities, understandings, and killings, that interesting happening known as aphasia is shunted onto a side track to be forgotten, as though it isn't really true, it doesn't really happen — surely not to us. Aren't we preferred outsiders?

But it happened to me. Why should aphasia be a disorder in disrepute which few want to examine intelligently, compassionately and realistically? Yet many would like to ignore it despite the tremendous, daily, unsung efforts of speech pathologists. Is it, in part, because too many aphasics do not regain the ability to speak readily or write? They do think and feel. Their thoughts and feelings must be conveyed somehow to those who will listen with their hearts as well as their heads.

A moratorium cannot be called on aphasia merely because it is a disorder not easily understood, one that doesn't lend itself to instant good results. If anything, the incidence of it may rise and with it the many paradoxes.

If aphasia clobbers someone in the field of medicine, someone able to spark real interest in this disorder among those who would ordinarily rise to his bait, chances are the medicine man finds himself unable to do what he so badly needs to for he is immersed in the very thing that is crying for his skill. To compound this initial overwhelming awfulness, having experienced aphasia he is given the non compos mentis name tag of *patient* and who, in the history of the world, has ever listened — really listened — to a patient?!!??

Is there a philosophical component to the reluctance on the part of many to wave the flag for aphasia? There seems to be reluctance on the part of those who in some way must deal with aphasics: physicians, nurses, physical therapists, pyschologists. How many more should be included? I don't doubt that they care, but can it be a truism that these same people do not want to be confronted with aphasia? Are there so few aphasics that the general public remains uninformed?

Perhaps the reluctance and disinterest, even fear lie in these few words: The brain is finite. The mind is infinite. Why should those eight words be so provocative? Many may not have given them substantive thought. We can explain the body and the brain. But is the reason for our existence simply a result of chance? Many of us, scientists included, resist that concept. One man (further information given upon written request), a Nobel Prize winner who has explored and dissected the brain for half a century, avers that the brain and the mind are separate and distinct. What makes us unique?

Here we are on a threshold which could lead to meaningful exploration, and yet if there weren't speech pathologists aphasics might be tossed in the discard bin. Is part of that sad condition because it is still impossible for many to separate the brain from the mind, with the grim consequence that in a final analysis, with many aphasics, no one is sure whether the damaged brain means much of the mind is gone?

Physical residuals can be dealt with for they can be seen. Inability to communicate via speech or to understand what is said is another matter, for what do those on the outside have to hang onto, those by the grace of God, not much cholesterol and no ballooning arteries, whom aphasia will never strike?

It is understandable, even to me, the reluctance many have in dealing with a disorder they do not comprehend. What I find well nigh impossible to understand is why all the ignoring? Why the difficulty in saying "we do not know"? Why the mask of absolute infallibility?

Aphasia often plays a discordant tune abhorrent to some and the patient feels a withdrawal from him by some of those in attendance whose behavior screams what they cannot bring themselves to say, "We're mad and we're cross and we say things we shouldn't because we don't know how to deal with aphasia. And we sure as heck don't understand you."

An aphasic may be bemused by some reactions he seems to provoke although he feels sure he has interpreted others correctly. Does the fact that he has been bereft of his ability to communicate normally give him, sometimes, an added insight into the outsiders who are confused because they are unable to project themselves into the tight spot from which he is trying to work his way out successfully?

Aphasia finds the mind struggling as it seeks ways to push a thought, one thought, any thought through a banged up brain to the world outside where it can be interpreted by other mortals not damaged by aphasia. Do these outsiders have the qualities of imagination and perception?

Think of the ways there are to communicate: speaking, signals, symbols, sounds, expressions, pantomime, drawing, writing — innumerable ways. The aphasic communicates in ways he hopes will be meaningful to those around him. The difficulty lies with his interpreters. Few persons have either the background or the training to unravel his train of thought, but those with imagination and considerable perception may find themselves quite adept in extracting his thinking.

Aphasia is frustrating beyond the telling of it. One minute oneself. In almost the twinkling of an eye he seems to others to be someone remote, strange, unable to talk in understandable language. In the light of my experience, the aphasic's mind is twirling and pirouetting from one thing to another as he is trying to assess the situation in which he finds himself plunged.

A mind trained in anything, in any subject, in any profession, business or work has a certain amount of facility, and it probably has never worked as hard as when aphasia uses that person as its target. A brain is damaged at strategic points. This does not prevent his mind from seeking, trying, devising ways to plod through an impenetrable road.

He wonders, "How do I tell them this? How pantomime for that? How can they be so dense? Why don't they really try to listen instead of distracting me by cupping their ears?" The aphasic (if he's like me) is grateful — oh so grateful — for his mate, his children and the speech therapist. He wonders how in the world does he rebuild a road out of rubble? How does he capture an elusive word long enough to write it or find an explosive that will push it through his hurt brain?

He feels the isolation by some — not that he is isolated from them but that they have isolated themselves from him. And he wonders, "What in heaven's name do they think has happened to me?" All this rejection because he cannot talk properly, normally, as he did before the accident? Accident! Probably in the making before he was born.

Every aphasic needs a family like mine and a perceptive speech therapist, but often there is a gaping difference between what he needs and what he has. He always needs support by family, speech therapist and friends, but, in common with everyone in trouble, the aphasic must learn to depend on himself and his private line to Universal Intelligence.

He must feel that aphasia is a challenge he can meet or it would not have been thrust upon him and that may be the biggest mountain of all. To scale it, he needs perseverance, patience, humor, insight in quantities he didn't dream he had. Any number of adjustments may have to be made depending on the severity of the stroke, family make-up, financial situation, and those things can add up to an enormously varied number of equations.

The aphasic may have to realign his life style and one imperative factor to remember is that we have to go from this point forward. It does no good to blame anything or anyone for the stroke, nor can we live on regrets. Recovery in any degree is based on positives: attitudes, motivations, utilizing intelligence well.

It sounds so easy! Challenges are rarely easy but they can be satisfying, stimulating, fun. To be a perpetual complainer surely must be one of the most abrasive, destructive attitudes one can have: demeaning to oneself; defeating to those subjected to it. A happy face, a kind word, loving thoughts are so much more rewarding to cultivate.

One of our friends of long standing has had rheumatoid arthritis for too many years. Right now she can neither stand nor sit for more than a whisper of time. Her marvelous sense of humor, her use of the choice ridiculous, the funny things she says make one forget the cruel pain she endures. Her moments of despair are almost always private; her conversation a tonic of laughter and wit. Like many an aphasic, she is sustained by the beauty she finds on the meadows of her mind.

What is it like in one's mind? If we are elastic enough to seek new ways when there seems to be no other route, we can find freedom unlike anything we've ever known or we can be in torment. Maybe it depends, in part, on how much imagination we can muster. It surely depends on how much personal security we have.

Ideas do not have to come only in packages of words we understand be they spoken or written. They can be plucked from the tree of knowledge, sifted through the sands of time, used as stepping stones criss-crossing the river of thought. We could be called idea-tasters. Whether one is interested in using his mind depends on him. Is that a difficult concept to envision?

In the beginning hours of aphasia, the moments when my mind went searching, asking and receiving, were moments of refreshment, of clarity, of truth glimpsed, of immanent peace. Can that be doubted even by thoroughbred skeptics no matter to what they choose to assign those feelings? I learned they belong to the province of the mind, an area largely uncharted by humans, a vastness covering eternity, whose vistas pour out in endless time, a pulsating excitement willing us to taste, to drink, to absorb, to learn.

With a jerk we are back to the present where reality tells us that in this century all too little has been accomplished in the field of aphasia. One sterling exception can be found in THE ACADEMY OF APHASIA and the knowledge and expertise of its members MUST be recognized, disseminated and used.

SOMEBODY PLEASE PLEASE PAY ATTENTION TO THIS NOISY APHASIC'S PLEA!!!

Still, aphasics arrive each day. But are they welcomed with, "We know we can help you" or "Oh, no, not another one of those!"

Some of us have found the mind a world enchanting.
Some may never discover a freshet of ideas.
But every aphasic must learn the feeling of being im-prisoned within himself.
And you —
All of you non-members —
You who stand locked out —
On which side would you rather be?

144

9

Reflections

Spring 1976

Time, in methodical progression, slips by on the wings of the wind and it is now six years post-stroke, the right distance for me to assess my feelings about aphasia today and the progress I think I have made.

How do I view my experiences with aphasia from this vantage point? Today the impact of aphasia is not as jarring as it was six years ago. I could only have written *Aphasia, My World Alone* while still immersed in the depths of aphasia simply because the passage of time obliterates much of the conscious impact of any experience. As I reread the material covered in my book I am swamped by a flood of memories which might have been buried in my unconscious had I not made the effort to dig them out and record them when they were close to the surface.

I have kept constructively busy and have been able to retrieve enough of my former business duties to feel a continuing partnership with my husband. And I find interest and delight in day by day occurrences: the antics of a family on a picnic in the park behind our home; a rare, lovely glimpse of a tiny boy using a bit of wadded up paper as a boat, floating it on water in a gutter, all the while talking to himself blissfully unaware of any world beyond the bounds of the one he is creating; the renewing beauty of bluebonnets, Indian paint brush and red clover necklacing roadsides along highways. All of these pleasures make boredom impossible.

Although the only aphasia I can discuss with intelligence is my own, the viewpoints of aphasics are needed. And I will comment on the following:

The importance of speech therapy.

The significance of the will of a patient in handling aphasia.

What I deem is my progress to date.

The Importance of Speech Therapy.

The approaches I learned from formal speech therapy have stood me in good stead since I've been on my own. I have been asked why I feel so strongly about the rewards of speech therapy and what do I think are the benefits to be gained through a professional speech therapist. Speech therapy and good rapport between the therapist and the patient were vital in my happy coping with a strange malady and I feel therapy should be started as promptly as possible.

It gave me:

Direction.

Discipline.

Planned assignments—short and varied.

Enthusiasm.

Philosophy.

Direction

It seems to me that the difference between professional help and lay help is in the objectivity of the professional in insisting that assignments be done, in knowing how to plan them best, and in asking for privacy without interruptions. I truly believe that the earlier one is encouraged to try to relearn accepted communication the easier will be progress. Speech therapy frees the patient from untold and untellable

146

worry about what he is to do. He is being helped by someone who knows and so he can bend all his energy, limited as it may be, to something concrete and purposeful – a valid reason for starting speech therapy early.

A speech therapist will help the patient avoid bad habits. For instance, I have had difficulty with *been* and *seem* turning into *benn* and *semm*. That is bad habit. It began after formal speech therapy had ended and using the typewriter had begun. When I realized that those two words were constant errors, I devised this scheme: I see them in my head as *bEEn* and *sEEm*. I shudder to think what bad habits I might have gotten into without professional help.

Rules give direction and are much better than any haphazard, hit-or-miss kind of program the patient might do on his own. A speech therapist can put the aphasic on the right path for further work to be done either by himself or with the help of lay people who have had instructions from the therapist. The patient needs rules about tackling his problems. Good rules and discipline bring good results.

Discipline

An aphasic patient has to realize that his ability to cope with living successfully is more important than how much of his loss is retrieved. The better he copes, the better adjustment he makes. The patient must never be allowed to give up on himself. The therapist can help him want to cooperate. And then, though it may be very, very slow progress, recovery in aphasia can be an ongoing process.

I am continually finding proof of that and I know that it only happens because of hard work. I still have to give my arm and leg instructions, but an important point is that now it takes less time to give orders which are responded to faster. Every day I exercise. And I do some of the following: invoice work, cross word puzzles, read, make phone calls, write letters, think about something, play games. The speech therapist helped me find out that to maintain progress I must discipline myself to doing some mental exercises every day – every single day. I still make comical errors: *Astoria, Oregon* was renamed *Ambrosia* and *Missoula, Montana* turned into *Macaroni.*

Planned assignments – short and varied

I did, and still do, best on short assignments and a variety of them. If variety is the spice of life, it may well be the way many aphasics function best. It works for me. I have x number of things to do. I begin with one and after working for a while I go on to something else, rotating until all the tasks are finished. By rotating and not sticking with the same job until it's done I can accomplish these things: each task seems easier; fatigue is less; everything seems interesting; frustration is minimal.

Enthusiasm

The speech therapist helps the patient feel excitement in making the slightest progress. It is easy for the patient to set unattainable goals for himself and the therapist is invaluable in helping him realize that progress is made in turtle steps. Smiles and touches do wonders. Happy laughing heals.

Philosophy

How an aphasic copes depends, in a nutshell, on how well he likes himself. The speech therapist may be the only one who can convey continually to the patient that the stroke has not altered his inner wholeness – the most important wholeness any of us has.

There are two subtle points that I feel bear discussion: the use of first names and the morale boosting of getting dressed. I am referring to the person who has just had a stroke and is in the hospital. My feeling is that to call a woman – of say 60 – Mary instead of Mrs. Brown may be defeating some of the positive impact of speech therapy before it has begun, because that could give the patient, especially an older one, the feeling that she is not a mature woman trying to cope. She is just a little girl. I think it is important for the aphasic patient to be made to believe she is capable of handling this latest blow by reason of her maturity. She might equate being called Mary with being considered a child who has no experience in living. Also, older people were taught never to call teachers by their first names (God Forbid) and if they are asked to call the speech therapist Peg or Harry that could mean what they are doing can't be serious work. I believe the first name bit makes a psychological impression and deserves discussion.

I am sure being helped to get dressed when the stroke was new had a salutary effect on my recovery. It was a procedure I never questioned. I'm glad I was up and at 'em in less than a week even though I spent much of that time lying down. In addition, I was encouraged to do things by myself, and it was literally months before I would let anyone do anything for me that I could do alone.

Certainly, instilling in an aphasic patient a sense of his own worth helps to create the most fortuitous atmosphere for getting better. The speech therapist has a golden opportunity for achieving that.

The Significance of Will

A letter from a family member of an aphasic contained this inquiry: "Where did your drive and determination originate – from within you? From others who encouraged? From their prodding? I doubt there are any simple answers. No simple answers for me or for anyone else. Rather, the answer may be a potpourri of many factors: genetic differences, body chemistry, the patient's self-image, the family's interest and understanding, the kind of damage that was done, the doctor's compassion and his wisdom in using another discipline, namely speech therapy, and the expertise of a speech therapist. Each summer my Alter Ego and I make trips to various parts of our country during which we have met aphasics and their families. From these journeys I have gleaned stories involving the will of an aphasic and I will tell about three of them.

Mrs. K is a wisp of a woman in her mid 70's who is badly aphasic but leading her usual get-after-'m-Gertie life with enthusiasm. She had a stroke eighteen months ago. There were minor physical residuals none of which are visible today. When she was dismissed from the hospital no speech therapy was on the agenda. I do not know whether this was because the family felt they couldn't afford it, or she had been in a hospital where it wasn't available, or her doctor felt it would not help and why spend money needlessly. However, she has a neighbor with the combination background of nursing and teaching who, although not too conversant with helping aphasics, plunged in with verve. They began to work while this teacher rooted around for competent, professional assistance. She found it through a program allied with the Visiting Nurse Association and now Mrs. K has speech therapy twice a week. She is making slow but real progress. She is a delight to watch. She attempts to say anything and is not embarrassed when the anything won't come. She is not disheartened by her fumbling efforts and uses body language to say her hearing is far from good.

She dearly loves working in her yard which she does every day of nice weather, enjoying her many varieties of flowers and her constant kitty companions. She does not tire easily. She has adjusted beautifully to the frustrations of aphasia. And why? My guess is that she has always coped well with the vagaries of living. The days when she was dependent on what we consider proper communication are behind her; much like a small boy and his "digging mud" she revels in digging in her yard with the beauty it ensures and the therapy it provides; she has understanding friends who bring her daily the trinity of joy and laughter and love and who come away from visiting her filled anew with her inward peace. I think it would never occur to Mrs. K to cope with any exigencies except as she does and with enthusiasm.

Then there's Mr. B, in his late 50's, the owner of a thriving business who was contended with his life and beginning to moderate his pace of living when suddenly came a massive stroke with many physical residuals and a good (or bad depending on your viewpoint) case of aphasia.

He worked right from the beginning with as much vigor as he could muster although he had fatigue to contend with. After six months his doctor and the therapists, speech and physical, told his family they had gone as far as they could. He would never be any better and, at that point, he wasn't significantly better than he'd been after having the stroke. His family was averse to accepting this verdict. Mr. B refused.

He is an intelligent man. He had built a successful business in the face of many challenges and he had met those efficiently. And he would meet this newest challenge in like manner. He tackled each area of disability with the same thoroughness, prodding and experimentation he had given to his business problems. The result? His doctor and the therapists are unbelieving. They said it couldn't be done. He had done it. His family is proud as punch but not too surprised. And Mr. B? Well, he isn't accustomed to being told "It can't be done." Today his walking is acceptable, he can use his right hand a little and his speech is limited but understandable. This may be a case of mind over matter. The moral surely is never to let a stroke patient give up on himself.

The third person is Miss Y, in her early 60's, whose stroke left her with right side residuals and aphasia. Her doctor indicated she needed no help with the aphasia since it wasn't too bad and would correct itself. It did not. Miss Y was sent, after hospitalization, to a convalescent home where she had a minimum of attention.

Getting her dressed was not encouraged since it was easier for those in charge to keep her in her nightgown. The physical therapist pumped her leg once a day and gave her a few exercises for her arm and hand. If she was helped to a wheel chair she was left in it two or three hours until she was crying with discomfort and fatigue. Miss Y grew very depressed. Her family, brothers and sisters and a favorite niece, would not listen to any other ideas. Their doctor said everything was being done that could be and they believed him implicitly. A year and a half went by with these dismal circumstances.

And then fate intervened on behalf of the patient. The home went into bankruptcy. Miss Y was moved to a well-run facility with a competent, gung ho staff, and lovely views: parks and children, lagoons and ducks, towering trees, snows in the winter and a profusion of flowers in the spring. She is receiving consistent therapies, both physical and speech; she dresses in the morning and undresses at night; she entertains company in a sunroom; she is no longer depressed. She feels she is getting help at last. Even her family members are impressed.

Why all those sorry months when she could have been helped? They were months when she was not encouraged to do anything by herself. Now she says she knows that one day she will be able to attend to her basic needs and get back to living by herself. And now she has the will to do it. Made possible, methinks, by the difference in the atmospheres of competence, beauty, and accomplishment which are surrounding her.

What is will? One apt definition the dictionary gives is that it is the power of choosing one's own actions. Suffice to say, it is a most important aspect in the recovery from a disorder as peculiar as aphasia with its propensity for making strange inroads into the communication system with which one is comfortable and used to having.

With aphasia, perhaps the patient longs for greener pastures elsewhere and uses his will to die; perhaps he feels there are still things to be done on this plane and uses his will to live; perhaps he is so completely and unhappily mixed-up that he becomes cantankerous, using his will to make those around him as miserable as he is. Of course, there's the grim possibility that the patient can't be meaningfully helped.

My thinking is that a lot of people feel as I do. The feeling is that it is useless to bemoan difficulties that befall us with repeated "Why did this happen to me? Why me?" Instead, how much better for us to think, even if we can't say, "Well, this *has* happened. Now what is the best way to tackle it?"

Aphasia has a plus sign when approached as a challenge rather than a disaster. As a challenge it means a more positive attitude, increases one's determination to get on top of this dumb happening, augments one's will to meet it head on. The result can be that everybody wants to do his best to help the aphasic regain some of his losses.

I plead for more understanding of the aphasic on the part of the medical and allied professions, an understanding which must be conveyed to the patient's family. In the final analysis, the *patient* determines how he will cope with his aphasia – a coping which will be materially helped or hindered by the attitudes, feelings and creativity of those best able to assist the aphasic: his family, speech therapist, and doctor.

My Progress to Date

One thing is obvious to me: my recovery continues. And that is important psychologically. I do not brood about things I cannot do such as willing my right hand to cooperate faster or being able to get the tops off jars, although I cannot deny there are moments when my inabilities are vexing. For instance, using the vacuum cleaner becomes increasingly difficult and therefore more annoying each time it is used.

The good part about not dwelling on what I cannot do easily is that one day I find that I can open a door with my right hand, or that doing invoices has become much easier since numbers are beginning to pop out at me without more than cursory hunting. One happy achievement came as I was searching on a map for a small town, not having an idea where it might be, and there it stood out as though it knew it had to push itself forward. That really was a first, and all by myself I whooped.

I will take various categories and show how I think I am progressing in those areas.

Speaking

Since having a stroke I have had the feeling – have it even now – that there is a stricture around my throat preventing speech. It's like talking against a current. Consequently, while my speech is greatly improved, it continues to be deliberate. My brain must be alerted as to what I am going to say, but the signals are given faster and responded to more quickly.

Errors I make in speaking can be comical. I meant to say to one of our sons, "Maybe your sister will iron that shirt." But what I said was, "Maybe your sister will mow that shirt." Sometimes they are reversals:

the word he used	*became*	the use he worded
that's what I do better		that's better what I do
Terry Farris,		Terry McFarris,
McAllen, Texas		Allen, Texas

Often errors mean getting the wrong word:

serialization	*became*	sterilization
biopsy		autopsy
codeine		cocaine
razor		raisin
confirmation		circumcision

At least errors can be said to add spice and make speech picturesque.

Reading

I am more thankful than I can say that I have regained my ability to read and comprehend the written word. And I do a great deal of reading, some fun and fluff, some exciting. Small print is not easy for me to zip through. The letters all tend to run together and, without a lot of concentration, what is before me are not words conveying an idea but a big jumble of specks. It's maddening and tiring.

The errors I made in reading add interest if not downright confusion. In this bunch of words I should have read, "How queer that a love of one's country should require defense." What I read with puzzlement was, "How love that a queer of one's country defense should require." Or this odd one: iron-on heat transfers *read as* iron-on heart transplants. Errors are often reversals involving single words:

revolution	*read as*	reluvotion
different		differenter

Errors happen less often than they did. Perhaps that is partly because reading is so much a part of my life that the more I do the easier it becomes. Remembering can be a problem. Not the simple facts of living like, "When is a dental appointment?" or "Where is some more toothpaste?" Those sorts of things don't seem to be much trouble. Neither is trivia that was delightful enough or interesting enough to be securely stuck in memory's bank.

The problem with remembering begins with ideas needing concentration to absorb. I can make a fairly intelligent comment on a specific idea shortly after reading it and temporarily digesting it. The difficulty is that I do not remember for long what the idea was or what I thought about it. I know that at the time I read it and discussed it I had found it stimulating. Maybe that's what counts: remembering how much fun those moments were and knowing I'm privy to them any time.

I also know that the only way I will remember that kind of material is to go over it every day, be refreshed on it constantly. Very much like exercises. To be effective they have to be done daily. And that may be one of the secrets of coping with aphasia: don't let up for a day. Keep doing whatever is helpful in making brain cells whirl meaningfully. Never give up. Repetitive practice is surely a key that helps an aphasic under the competent direction of a speech therapist. The practice often has to be maintained a long, long time.

Writing

Although I use only my left hand for typing that does not preclude my attending to lively and interesting correspondence. My book has brought me delightful letters from many corners of our world and I have appreciated the thoughtfulness prompting those letters. Answering them is an activity I relish.

One of the most pertinent comments I have received is this: "Thanks to your book I am confirmed in my belief that the person is *still there* behind the disability." Bless that writer for her perspicacity.

Writing jells my thinking. It is like a jigsaw puzzle requiring organization and thought until the words fall where they belong. For me, writing entails the constant use of a dictionary and a thesaurus for correct spelling and for hunting to find a word. The fact that I'm likely to forget both the spelling and the word doesn't bother me unduly. At least I have the resources in which to locate them again.

Those resources are also great for doing cross word puzzles which are good tools for giving the ole bean a workout. And there are other games which involve writing. When my brothers and I were children, our mother had pads of the game shown on p. 155 printed for us, and we and our friends spent a lot of time thinking up weird categories and unusual key words. The ones I use make playing the game fairly simple.

Key Word	BIRDS	FLOWERS	TREES	ANIMALS	COUNTRIES
T					
R					
A					
I					
L					

Another writing game is finding words within another word. For example:

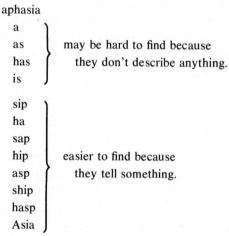

aphasia

a
as
has
is
} may be hard to find because they don't describe anything.

sip
ha
sap
hip
asp
ship
hasp
Asia
} easier to find because they tell something.

Naming the states and their capitals is another brain twirler. These are helpful games for aphasics who are able to manage them. Vegetating idleness is to be avoided. Thinking idleness is stimulating and can be creative.

Business

Business details I like. They can be done at home which means there is no problem about getting to and from the office and there are not the sorts of interruptions there always seem to be in an office. I enjoy checking invoices, determining how our accounts are being shipped, which need to have follow up, what kinds of direct orders we are getting and from whom. There are a myriad of things needing attention.

Market weeks, with their attendant confusion, are not manageable. Working with a customer is beyond my abilities. Discussing the selling points of garments, displaying the samples for the buyer, writing an order while being aware of any comments the customer may make, and doing all these things at once? NO. Indeed, I may never again be ready for it.

Working behind-the-scene details at home by myself at my own pace is rewarding. Numbers, even long ones, are easier to locate on an order than they were. Consequently, invoices are dispatched faster. Most things are done with my left hand and, although my right hand is far from a total loss, it still has to be told what to do and doing whatever takes it so miserably long that impatience tells me to save my innards aggravation by using my left hand. I continue to write checks with my left hand and sign them with my right. Even so, that right hand sometimes clamps and I must pry it from the pen, shake it, rub it, do a few exercises and begin again.

Fatigue

No longer do I experience the drowning fatigue that plagued me for 3 years post-stroke. While I realize there are quickly met limits beyond which I must not venture, I am not swatted daily by unremitting fatigue. I tire most easily as a result of simultaneous stimulation from more than one source. For instance, if we are watching television and someone tells me something the chances are that nothing registers from either source. And the resulting confusion is tiring. It is easy, too easy, for me to lose the right channel. Now if I know someone is going to talk to me while the television is blaring, or if I am in a group of people, the strategy I use is to consciously tune out everything but one person and concentrate on what he is saying. It does work. It is enormously fatiguing.

Fatigue is also a part of locating products in a super market or items in a department store. And trying to buy clothes. Not long ago we went to a shop where my husband had heard I could easily find what I wanted. When we got there we found that he had to wait in a foyer while I shopped. I wonder if you nonaphasics have any idea of the feeling that assails me in that kind of a situation. It is a cousin to panic and I can't cope. Except that I know I will cope. On that occasion I used the blocking out technique and came home with two additions to my wardrobe – a triumph which counteracted the fatigue.

If I do too much (too many invoices at one time), or have too much stimulation of any kind (lots of company all at once), I have learned that fatigue in toto is apt to follow. Ergo, I have a built-in excuse for not doing whatever it is I decide I shouldn't or don't want to do. I now can say NO without the slightest twinge of guilt to a telephone caller who wants me to collect for a drive. I rest on past laurels.

Lately, my appetite has been improving. Diet must have much to do with fatigue. Actually, I am much, much better. One lesson I have learned: I realize beyond a doubt that my life must be restricted if I am to continue feeling well.

Decisions

The one major decision I have made was to decide I would no longer drive. Deliberately I let my driver's license expire. When the time came to renew it we learned that I would have to take a behind-the-wheel test which I would not do, my reason being that if I were the officer giving the test I would not pass me. For any number of reasons I know I should not drive. If I were unhappy with the sort of isolation not driving metes, the situation might have been that I would have taken the test and sheer determination might have insured passing. Doesn't it boil down to how one assesses priorities?

When anything major needs to be done to the house my husband decides, selects, and supervises. I enjoy. For example, two years ago we had the entire house carpeted. He was here. Lately, a project has been reglazing the bathtubs and he has insisted it be done when he could be on hand. I find it a very comfortable arrangement.

Shopping I'm apt to do via the telephone in lieu of hopping from store to store. Telephoning is still not one of my favorite pastimes but it's much less wearing than crowds of people and merchandise. Unless I'm totally bereft of ideas, I usually call in an order for a wedding gift or items I need and so far it has worked out well.

Restaurant dining is pleasurable providing noise level is minimal. Reading a menu and deciding what I would like is more fun than it was and usually My Dear conveys my order to the waiter. The good part is that I now feel more confident of my ability to handle that kind of situation and know I won't be tossed into a deciding tizzy if my selection is not available.

Sometimes we have dinner company at home and there can be confusion in entertaining. Getting as much as possible ready beforehand, which means almost everything, helps when guests arrive and chitchat begins. Lots of talking and extra people trying to help can lead to my not knowing what is happening or where anything is or what I should be doing. And I have to keep a tight grip on myself. Also, it is not easy for me to eat and be expected to converse. I try to get others to do the talking. However, entertaining has become an experience I can manage with considerable ease providing there has been proper planning and organization.

Decisions I have had time to mull over are not bothersome. The troublesome ones are those that must be made on the spur of the moment, as in a telephone call when the salesperson says, "We don't have any more of that color. What other color do you want?" When I'm caught off guard, which happens occasionally, my decision making mechanism takes a roller coaster double loop leaving me in a frantic empty place and I may not answer intelligently. My decisions demand organization and discipline if I want to avoid feeling *non compos mentis*.

People

I like people in small doses. There is one group I should like to be a contributing part of, having been a member for many years, but the meetings are beyond my ability to enjoy as I did pre-stroke. I cannot separate conversations and, without tremendous concentration, what I hear is a cacophony of noise. Today I spent much more energy and effort listening than I did pre-stroke. And I was trained to listen. One learns how much useless chatter there is, my own included, with "you know" and "I mean" thrown in every few words. It makes one pause and wonder. There may come a time in our people society when speech as we know it may no longer be necessary. Maybe it will be mind-to-mind conversation without the inane drivel we spout in today's world. Of course, there's always the chance that internal nonstop chatter might be worse. But maybe there will be a day when aphasics won't have to worry about being understood. Happy, happy maybe!

Telephone

It can be said truthfully that my feelings about the telephone are ambivalent.

It is not as hard as it was to give information over the phone: addresses, phone numbers, charge plate numbers, and items desired. However, I find that when I must relate information about our four lines of merchandise to my traveling mate I'm apt to get breathless. I must be careful not to reverse numbers and if I haven't a written list of everything I need to tell him there are sure to be some things I forget or names that I can't remember.

Names are a nemesis. For example: Hans had left a walkie-talkie plugged in and it was on a radio/record player. I needed to ask him if or when it should be unplugged, but I hadn't written it. Now, how do I ask him over the phone when I cannot think of what it is called or how to explain plugging in or where the whatever is sitting?

Talking with those nearest and dearest to me is fine. Friends too. Reporting important items accurately or making quick decisions can be exhausting.

Exercise

The exercises I have done following the stroke have kept my right arm and shoulder fairly limber and I have learned they must be done every day if their effectiveness is to be maintained. If, for whatever reasons, they are tossed aside for a few days stiffness sets in and getting them started again is doubly hard. I have a stationary bicycle and I try to ride it two miles a day which takes care of my leg.

The leg is not too much trouble even with no bicycling. There are times when my walking is almost normal and there are times when I have a definite limp. When walking is more than a long block or I'm trying to walk fast or it is cold then my right leg tightens, acts like a wooden appendage and drags. In cold weather my right arm tightens, too, seems like a tinker toy stuck on me askew and has to be manipulated to become a semifunctioning part of me.

I have devised my own routines for exercising and usually spent 20–25 minutes not including bicycling. Counting must be done in my head, otherwise I'm apt to find I'm doing nothing but counting. With my aphasia there seems to be something about saying things out loud which preempts anything else I am doing. Perhaps it's tied in with the doing one thing at a time syndrome. I cannot think about other things while I'm exercising, and closing my eyes helps me to concentrate. And unless I really concentrate I find myself doing the same exercise over and over while I'm daydreaming. Bicycling, while staying in one spot, is the only activity during which I can roam in my mind anywhere I please.

A soak in the tub first makes exercising easier. For me there is no satisfactory substitute for a hot tub bath, but I am aware that even a couple days of feeling "poorly" can make getting in and out (especially out) a major chore. And that makes the danger of falling more acute. A shower chair has been found to be a respectable compromise between sitting in the tub and standing under the shower.

Well, there are times when we have to accept compromises and use our imaginations to make them as palatable as possible. Teetery-tottery days make me appreciate compromise. They also force me to realize that, no matter how I feel, exercising is vital to maintaining the right amount of suppleness in order to live in reasonable comfort.

Noise

Mondays can be tired days after a week-end of games blaring from the t.v. The effect of constant, unpleasant-to-me noise – people yelling, music blasting, a barrage of raucous clanging – has a deleterious impact on my innards. Grating, bombastic noise can be ungluing.

And yet, sounds can be soothing: a solitary mocking bird within eye range giving a virtuoso musical performance; the wind – a gentle, caressing breeze or a wild, enthusiastic roar; the chirp of crickets; the sleepy lull of mourning doves; the laughter of children. Those are healing sounds.

Pain

It is odd to me that pain seems exaggerated since having the stroke. What I was accustomed to shrugging off now causes more discomfort than it did once upon a time. But, there it is. Without regular exercises I would be as supple as a broomstick and moving any part of me would be miserable. Headaches are now at a minimum and there I hope they stay. Does one really have to have a lot of pain to realize how beautiful life can be without it? And oh joy and happy hours! I have been free of completely debilitating headaches for six months. No wonder I feel renewed.

Housework

It seems paradoxical that when I find my home so enjoyable I also find attempting to keep the house in some kind of order a point of monumental frustration. And yet, for me, that schism is understandable.

The helper we have had for many years now comes only occasionally. I find the thought of breaking in someone else a chilly one and we continue to hump along as best we can. Housekeeping, per se, has been an activity I have avoided if possible. Until I was married it was a department I knew little about and during the forty years since I have known much more than I could savor gracefully. The truth is that all of it bores me to distraction.

Worse still, it hurts. There are spots in my back that scream when I've done even a little activity like sweeping or making a bed, and because I'm still tied to the one thing at a time routine I cannot soar to higher places as I scrub and be assured of getting anything accomplished. It is frustrating to try to do housework largely with one hand and to find things that need doing for which I haven't the strength – things like opening a window or getting something to or from the top shelf of the linen closet.

This harangue doesn't mean I'm not eternally grateful that I can do as much as I can. Rather, I think it indicates that since housework was never one of my favorite activities the stroke made it even less appealing. As for cooking, I do whatever needs to be done. And how lucky I am to have a mate who enjoys fixing all kinds of foods. He is great with fish, steak, hamburgers, turkey, sweetbreads; can get a meal ready quickly; and when he is freer to experiment he will probably be an honest to goodness gourmet cook.

Summary

The quiet life has many advantages. I enjoy being surrounded by the things I like best: the rooms in our home; our storytelling pictures; the changing view of the lake; the glorious sunsets; and books. I am not lonely, although I'm frequently alone. Time with my mate of four decades is wonderfully satisfying. It is interesting to watch grown-up children in their various stages of development and they can always be reached by phone. So can friends. There is contentment in living on my terms.

Because I have improved markedly, many people think I have made a complete recovery. They are not apt to notice my thumb which insists on turning in and can be held straight only when I concentrate hard on getting it so. Funny that a simple activity like putting on hand lotion means contending with a thumb that's always in the way. And friends don't see me getting dressed after a bath, only to find my right side is still soggy because I've forgotten to dry one side of me that doesn't feel wet. They certainly can't look inside my head during moments when I'm fumbling around trying to get out of one of those empty spaces. There are lots of little things my friends do not know but it's a game to keep them in the dark. The important thing is that I don't fib to myself. And I do know that my recovery is an ongoing process.

Conclusions

At this distance of six years from the onset of my aphasia and in view of my experiences with aphasics from other parts of our land, I feel more strongly than ever about the merits of speech therapy and its value in giving the aphasic tools for continuing therapy when he is on his own. The importance of speech therapy cannot and must not be minimized.

For those taking care of aphasics I plead for the kind of understanding that goes beyond accepted ideas of the norm; for insight that reaches out in words and thoughts to those deep levels each of us has; for viable programs geared to teaching the patient how to tackle retrieving his losses. Truly, an aphasic needs to be surrounded by optimism and confidence and by the compassion which gives him that stabilizing sense of his own worth.

As for the progress of one aphasic – me: The more I am aware of the small but significant things in my life – a single rose – a butterfly on a window sill – the antics of a kitten – indeed, the more I am attuned to the vibrancy all around me, the better am I able to adjust to and delight in living.

Once, I enjoyed tramping on our acreage, walking through its shadowy woods, wandering along its picturesque ravines. Today, my strolls are carefully calculated ones where the dangers of falling are minimal and I can stop in sight of my Fisherman to savor a lift of the spirit as I drink in the blue of the sky, the roll of a hill, the birds by the water.

Physically, my life is quite circumspect. Mentally, I am finding freedom I never seemed to have time to investigate pre-stroke and I am excited about the challenges I find therein. Each day brings new discoveries. Each day is a moment to enjoy and I deem it a laughable moment when I turn *panorama,* a word of lovely connotations, into *paranoia.*

And so, six years post-stroke find me busy, continually retrieving bits of abilities lost to a stroke with aphasia, and contented to live a circumspect but full life.

Spring 1977

I am a recovering aphasic. I think I will always be a recovering aphasic. One day my life made a turn of 180 degrees. It was a busy, active, happy life. I was involved in many projects, managed our office, took care of our children and kept the home fires burning. It is still a busy, active, happy life. ONLY *busy* and *active* have entirely new meanings, new dimensions. The office is out; the children are up and gone – tho not too far; projects are like writing this which appeals to me and actually is therapy; business details are done at home by me at my pace; and oh what wonderful ideas there are for anyone to capture – anyone like me who has time to enfold these elusive, fragile marvels. It has been a gratifying transition.

In this rearranged pattern of living, my husband and I have met lots of aphasics from many parts of our land. Those have been fruitful experiences. The areas I will discuss seemed of real import to many of those aphasics. And those things are:

The early rememberings of some aphasics.

Myths of aphasia.

That dreadful fatigue.

Hallelujah for team work.

The Early Rememberings of Some Aphasics

The early hours of aphasia! For some of us strange and wonderful: the cadence of the immediate felt as thru a soft mist; unearthly beauty tingling; a keen awareness of eyes, of looks, of tones. There was a breath-taking look at a cosmic pattern into which I fit; there was a lasting knowing of how beautiful is the step from this plane to the next; there was my total awareness of those around me; of their gestures, their expressions, the words they used, what they said, the tones of their voices, the way they touched me; and there was an insight into how I would be handled, how I could expect to be treated, what those around me thought of me and how they reacted to my ailment.

Do you suppose that some of the depression associated with aphasia is due to thoughtless things said within earshot of the patient in the early hours of illness. I wonder. I, and there are many others, have never been more acutely aware than in the first few days of aphasia. And that awareness happened in fleeting moments. If a patient feels he is surrounded by confident, positive people, then he begins to feel confident and positive himself. It is the negative, uncertain, unsure attitude he has read that is damaging. Those early, vital bits of understanding are surely important in helping or hindering an aphasic's ability to cope successfully with aphasia.

But do aphasics discuss these early feelings? According to those with whom I have discussed this, the answer is usually NO. The reasons given were: Nobody ever asked them what they remembered; when they were ready to be dismissed from the hospital, they still could not communicate well enough to try; they knew that if they did express their feelings about their initial insights, they would have been treated like children having fantasies. One voluble aphasic put it this way, "I finally learned that it was foolish to rock the boat or I might never get out of this 'jail' and I was tired of having them think I didn't have good sense."

There are some of us who did try to tell of these early experiences which had been so amazing, so revealing, but it was usually to our sorrow. It is not conducive to happy coping with aphasia when the patient is made to feel he is not telling the truth, those things could not have happened, aphasics never remember. Who says so? Whoever has really bothered to find out?

One woman, who had a stroke and aphasia many years ago, felt she should tell her doctor how inspiring had been her first few hours of this odd disorder. She told him. His reply? "Oh, don't be silly. You couldn't have remembered." She says the clarity of those moments has been a sustaining force in her life ever since then.

Another aphasic spoke of these initial revelations as though he were an observer. He described himself as being completely detached, watching with interest and acute awareness what was happening to him and what were the reactions of others. And amazed, even then, how little emotional involvement he felt.

There are aphasics who, in all probability, will never consciously remember anything about the first few days. But there are a number of aphasics who have felt this early total awareness and deemed their experience such a personal one that they were reluctant to tell anybody. Rather, they hugged those moments to themselves in awe that they should have been privy to them. Please do not assume that every aphasic does not recall early happenings. The answer may be that he cannot tell of them or he does not want to, either because he is unwilling to risk ridicule or his rememberings are too special to be shared.

Think on these things. Professionals can be such a marvelous force in helping the aphasic learn to cope well with a traumatic disorder.

Myths of Aphasia

If ever there was a malady where insights need to be shared, it is aphasia with its peculiar ramifications. One thing gleaned from fellow aphasics is their annoyance with the number of myths that surround aphasia. Aphasics can expound for hours about these. Naturally it takes hours since a lot of us cannot talk fast. Here are examples:

If the patient appears comatose, he will not hear anything, and if he should hear he will not understand, and if he should understand he will not remember.

The patient does not understand anything that is said to him so it is all right to talk about him. Even say he is never going to be any better than he is right now.

The aphasic will not remember, so it is o.k. to say almost anything in his presence. Tactless words? He will not remember them.

All aphasics are sorta kooky anyway.

Speak loud. The patient cannot talk and does not seem to understand so he must be hard of hearing. (Truth is, sounds often become the most horrendous kind of noise and can be very distressing to the aphasic.)

He said that word yesterday. There is no reason why he cannot say it today.

Aphasia destroys the thinking, whole person. (And that is probably the unkindest cut of all.)

Perhaps these are myths only to the patient. Would any intelligent person believe these statements always had substance in fact? Yet, why do many aphasics feel they have been subjected by professionals to the sorts of prejudicial attitudes the above examples represent? Is it because there is little viable communication between the professionals, the patient, and his family? Is everyone too busy? Is there simply too much to be done?

Unfortunately, remiss omissions and commissions happen too often even in the best of hospitals. The examples I will give occurred in big hospitals where there should have been superior help, sensible advice, intelligent treatment, and tools for understanding aphasia. They relate to misunderstandings about aphasia and/or indifference to the aphasic and his family.

One aphasic was scolded constantly because she complained of being tired. Certain it is that the scolders could not imagine the blanketing, overwhelming, drowning fatigue of aphasia. In the presence of the aphasic, a neurologist told the wife that the patient would never be more than a vegetable and should be put in a nursing home for custodial care. The wife was frantic because she knew the patient was understanding what was being said. And he was. With horror. The postscript to this is that the patient is not a vegetable and in a few months was back at work.

A prominent man in a community had a stroke with aphasia, a disorder neither he or his wife knew much about. He was given token help in therapies, both physical and speech. Not once did anyone give his wife even a clue as to what was going on, what could be expected, how she could manage best this situation, how she could begin to understand it. No one queried her about her husband nor were her questions answered except with evasions.

The daughter of an aphasic (and he is badly aphasic) felt deeply that the man she had always known was intact behind his disability. It would have been comforting and reassuring to her if one of the professionals had reinforced that belief. But no one did. The reinforcement came from another aphasic. And it is a happy knowing for them both: pleasant for the daughter and an inestimable help to her father who knows that she knows that inside he is o.k.

True stories these. And they show how easy it would have been to avoid the unhappiness they brought. In no way does this recital mean that we of THE CLUB do not appreciate the wealth of material being circulated among those who have prime care of aphasics. Or the efforts made on our behalf to understand better a strange disorder and make it more palatable to those who confront it, and to their families who must learn to live with it.

Is it possible that no one is reporting officially these sorts of misunderstandings? Very possible. Sadly, the longer an individual continues to make an error in judgment, the deeper the error becomes entrenched until, suddenly, it is a "fact." Maybe that is behind the myths about aphasia. If thinking, observations, and insights are shared, mistakes in understanding should be alleviated.

That Dreadful Fatigue

Fatigue is an aftermath of aphasia affecting almost all persons who are aphasic. We have heard about it constantly from the many aphasics we have met in our travels. One man said, "It's a bad, bad tired. Bad. Very bad." Another aphasic explained it like this, "All my parts are tired. Can't eat. Can't think. Can't do anything. It's awful." How true! A woman summed it up thusly, "It's not like any tiredness I've ever had. I didn't know there could be such tiredness. It's total. And nobody – just nobody – understands."

I was plagued by dreadful fatigue. Often those who have a lot of energy have difficulty understanding why an aphasic should be so unreasonably tired. I had bunches of energy pre-stroke. I have had precious little of it since. Omitting emotional reasons which are numerous, there are two whys for the fatigue that descends on many aphasics. These are reasons to which, perhaps, too little attention has been given. One is the inordinate amount of cerebral activity aphasia necessitates. The other is nutrition.

Unless one has been immersed in aphasia or is an astute speech therapist, it is almost impossible to comprehend how much cerebral activity is necessary for the simplest task to be accomplished or the most rudimentary sentence spoken. And that kind of wrestling continues and can be handled successfully only when the aphasic knows he must discipline himself to wrestling with it every forever day of his life. This is a fact many aphasics face and probably it is best if they reach that realization themselves. If they have been disciplined to working daily at retrieving some of their losses, they can come to that conclusion with some grace. But if someone bombards them with that bit of serious stuff early in aphasia, it could be terribly defeating.

Do you ever remember having to consciously tell a hand to pick up a piece of paper and how to do it? A foot to step over a twig along the path? Give directions to an uncooperative body on how to get up from sitting on the floor? Determine just how one does put on a pair of pants? Try again and again to construct, remember, and say a simple complete sentence? Being unsure of what was said to you although you were right there listening the whole time? Wonder how to climb out of that blank area in your head – not just a quiet spot but an empty, nonfunctioning, nonthinking, nothing place?

And do you realize how much energy the aphasic may have to expend to accomplish any task: for instance, taking a bath and getting dressed? New pathways can be made in his brain but unless they are used constantly, the paths may soon be obliterated. Truly, it behooves everyone to realize that the fatigue many aphasics complain about and succumb to is very, very real.

It is now almost seven years since I had a stroke and, although it takes less time to give instructions to various parts of me and those orders are met faster, the instructions still must be given consciously or the intended action does not get done. Take a simple act like putting the date on a check to be written and at the same time thinking about the amount of the check. The result often is that my hand is poised over the date space but nothing gets written. And I sit wondering why.

Even today I seem to have to direct my whole attention to accomplishing one task at a time where I once could juggle several easily. For example, if I am using the adding machine, I must concentrate solely on the figures to be added and never wander my mind as to what those figures represent. This I have found too: I can use my right hand to punch the adding machine, except that it means telling fingers the key to press which means I am no longer concentrating on what the number is and am apt to make errors. Therefore, I have found it easier, less wasteful of my limited energy, if I use my left hand to work the adding machine while using my right to follow the list of numbers. That way my right hand is involved in one movement only: just sliding from one number to the next.

There is always fatigue. But in the circumspect life I lead, the fatigue is manageable. And, considering the extraordinary amount of cerebral activity necessary if I am to function adequately, my present milieu is the best for me.

And then there is nutrition. Methinks a dietician should be a viable spoke in the wheel of competence surrounding the patient. Diet may be another aspect of the patient's life where there must be change.

Certainly his whole life pattern is subject to careful scrutiny and diet ought to be a part of it.

When the patient is in the hospital, the dietician plans meals with that particular patient in mind. But does anyone check to see whether or not meals have been eaten by the patient? And if not much is being eaten, does anyone find out why? Is anything done to correct it? Surely there are things that could be done to relieve this kind of troublesome situation. Any of you familiar with small children will have learned that when too much food is piled on a plate, it often turns a child completely from eating. The same thing happens with some aphasics. Me included. Although the patient is weary and really does not see how he can eat, he knows he needs some sustenance. But the sight of a lot of food can be sickening. Everyone is not plumb devoted to eating. You may say there is nothing that can be done. I say there has to be a way. Are smaller portions and fruit drinks between meals an unreasonable request?

And then I think it is imperative that the dietician see that the patient and his family are given the sort of diet to be followed – given specifics. Food does not have to be complicated to be effective and the more the aphasic is involved in preparing it, the simpler it better be. This is an area where disciplining oneself to eat properly can be difficult. A prize example is the writer: I am alone fairly often; food is not too interesting; meal-getting is now a bore; and I am addicted to sweets.

Nutrition is a subject on which there should be active communication between the staff, the dietician, the patient and his family if there is to be understanding of the aphasic's needs. And if something constructive is to be achieved to meet them. It goes without saying that good nutrition is of prime importance in recovery from anything and it should help, surely, to eliminate some of the overriding fatigue assailing lots of aphasics.

Hallelujah for Team Work

Ideally, the best approach to the care of aphasics is through team work. It can be presumed that team members know a great deal about aphasia and its pervasive effects, but how regularly do those team members discuss their thinking and insights with other people of their own persuasion or those who make up the team? After meeting and listening to aphasics from many places, one wonders if the team discusses those insights at all. They seem to be discussed seldom with the patient's family and almost never with the patient. So, if not shared, what good do those insights accomplish? It is true, in a different context, that aphasia can be as frustrating to nurses and other professionals as it is to the patient. All the more reason for staff members to discuss each situation if they are to make an intelligent assessment on how to handle the aphasic.

A stroke wing is desirable. Then the nursing staff does not have a potpourri of ailments to attend to but is revved up mentally to care for stroke patients. Which brings up another point: the staff does have to know more about the aphasic than sex, age, and where the lesion is. And because one aphasic has a certain disability and acts in a certain way, no one can expect every other aphasic to react in like manner. Frankly, aphasics need those who are blessed with imagination, to whom the word innovation means creativity, who are not bound by rule 15 on page 102.

In aphasia the patient watches and listens, and the team members learn they must if a particular patient is going to be handled to fit his particular needs. And probably the only trait fitting all aphasics is that their communication mechanisms have blown a bunch of fuses. Interested watching yields many rewards. Eyes tell so much.

The other day I heard about a woman who has been an aphasic for several years and only recently began to be able to read simple sentences. It points up the fact that for many aphasics recovery is ongoing provided the aphasic is continually plugging. It does not just happen. The aphasic needs encouragement for the slightest advance – maybe even the slightest effort. And a team can give him that encouragement. Give it daily and lots of it. Hopefully, this kind of buoying up will last when the aphasic no longer has a team to depend on. Temper, depression, anger, and frustration sometimes evolve as tenacity and determination.

A team is a wonderful thing if it is really made to function. It should not be a perpendicular, totem-pole arrangement with every member feeling that his discipline should be top dog. The team ought to be thought of as a wheel with each discipline a spoke and the patient at the hub. The result should be that the patient learns to cope well with his disability. The team members must know how to communicate with each other, learn as much as they can about each patient, discuss the treatment a particular patient is getting, and decide upon the best procedures to follow to benefit the patient most. And discuss these things with his family. Nor should the patient be kept in the dark.

It is important to realize that, for many aphasics, early impressions of staff have lasting results. Expressions in eyes. Tones of voices. Words that are said. These right-after-stroke impressions can materially help or hinder the patient's ability to cope. In essence, they rebound to the staff who made those impressions. If they made the patient feel he is surrounded by wise people who have confidence in themselves and in him, he is apt to react by doing as well as he can which in turn makes the staff feel successful. Excellence mushrooms. And that is good. Professionals must remember that their challenge with the aphasic patient is to return him to his home as a comfortable family member. And to help his family learn to be comfortable with aphasia.

The team approach is fine. It is not always effective. Disciplines sometimes do not work well with each other. This is one time when they must if their goal is helping the patient get the maximum of benefits. Those benefits will be long-lasting ones felt by the patient, his family, and the staff. Like interest, the benefits accrue to everyone's advantage. Enthusiasm and a sense of humor are great catalysts in difficult times. And why not try for the best?

One thing can be counted on: Aphasics everywhere will cheer for the team, try by remote control to inspire the team, will be happy for the successes of any team. And they will give the team their blessings every day – every single day.

Summer 1977

Ten Important Reminders Regarding Aphasia
For Speech Therapists
1. Remember that no matter what deficits the aphasic has, his inner wholeness is intact.
2. Remember the psychological benefits to the patient and the therapist when an aphasic is considered a mature, thinking adult.
3. Remember to let the aphasic decide which of his deficits are most important to him, and where he wants to concentrate.
4. Remember that multiple disciplines are rarely handled successfully by an aphasic, especially in the beginning. The patient must choose.

171

5. Remember that each aphasic is different and needs therapy designed for him alone.
6. Remember that an aphasic is more apt to keep trying when his retraining has been laced with enthusiasm, excitement, laughter and love.
7. Remember that text book learning and examples are guidelines only. Each aphasic is a new challenge worthy of creative therapy.
8. Remember that the aphasic needs tailored directions to use when on his own. Therapy may last forever.
9. Remember that enormous amounts of energy and cerebral activity are necessary in retrieving losses. Ergo: Fatigue besets many aphasics.
10. Remember to help an aphasic realize that the quality of his life is more important than how much of his disability is repaired.

Spring 1978

My aphasia is forever. What does that mean? And why should I, a "recovered" aphasic, say that? One dictionary definition of recovery is that it is a return to soundness. But I am not as sound as I was pre-stroke 8 years ago. And I never will be.

Now progress is an upbeat word and I have made progress —lots of it. I work daily at exercising, both physical and mental. And I am convinced that consistent working at this retrieval makes it possible for me to maintain the progress I have made. And here and there make a little more. It is certainly healthier for aphasic me to concentrate on progress and not waste precious energy thinking, wanting, expecting complete recovery tomorrow, next week, or sometime soon. Better, too, to use effectively the abilities that remain and not mourn over those that were lost.

Not many of us who have been initiated into aphasia have had any idea of what aphasia is or what it will mean to us. We find ourselves floundering in a sticky morass and we need help to climb out. Sometimes we reject the help that is proffered. But please listen! The aphasic has had a devastating blow. His communication circuits are jammed. He's met an impasse. His life is at a crossroads. No matter what his reactions are, he has an overwhelming need for direction; for being considered a mature, thinking person; for encouragement; for loving touches; for happy smiles. How well he will cope depends a great deal on how easily and constantly he is given these necessities.

When do we decide how we will cope with our aphasia? When do we realize that it is going to be a companion the rest of our lives? Twice I came to grips with this peculiar happening. The first time was right after I had had an arteriogram – when I knew that I was going to be on this plane a while longer and the best thing to do was to get busy and work as hard as I could to resolve this whatever it was. I knew there had to be lots of hard work ahead of me – no miraculous cure. But, at that point, my thinking was on an hour to hour basis – always in the present, not geared to what I would be doing in a month, much less 8 years.

The second insight came when the stroke was several weeks old. We're not sure of the exact time. On this occasion my husband, Hans, told me he had seen the arteriogram and that the left side of my brain was a complete blank. In my imaginative, unscientific way I concluded that meant that after more than half a century a whole new set of paths would have to be made in my brain – paths for ideas to get through, for words to be found and spoken, for sentences to be properly arranged, for understanding what was said to me, for reading and writing – new paths for anything relating to communication. And that meant continuous work to keep those paths clear or they would soon be impassable. That meant REAL challenge. I never questioned the rightness or wrongness of my thinking. I just knew that my aphasia was forever. Progress I could make. Total recovery was not possible.

Aside from the damage, it seems to me that coping with aphasis depends largely on three factors.

How we feel about ourselves.

The reactions of our family.

The quality of help accorded to us by professionals.

How We Feel About Ourselves

I have been asked many times what motivated me to work hard – to have an optimistic attitude. One answer to that is found in the far long ago. I was comfortable with my parents, my brothers, delighted in my home and my life. My mother and father gave me the tools for learning anything, never dented my curiosity, greeted ideas no matter how peculiar with interest. They gave me the feeling that life was a splendid adventure full of problems to be solved by a mind honed to problem solving. My father told me just before I was married that nothing would ever happen that I couldn't manage. Amazed I was. But, as always, I believed him.

How much did my early years have to do with my motivation? Immeasurably much. I have always liked being me. Now, had my background been different, my marriage rocky, my attitude about myself more crummy than nice – well, then my reactions following a stroke could have been anything but positive. I think, truly, that a major force in motivation is how well the aphasic likes himself – how secure he is. And how important it is to him to recoup some communication losses.

The Reactions of Our Family

My husband, right from the start, has handled me with patience, intelligence, interest, and love. He never once acted as though something was dreadfully amiss – as though I had changed. He treated me with the same consideration and tenderness I was accustomed to having from him. He has been more protective than he was and has run interference for me when things got a little out of hand – things like a social function or a business hassle. He has encouraged me to do anything I felt I could do and some I was not sure I was ready to tackle. And he has applauded my writing.

Our youngest was nearly 19 at the time I had the stroke which means our four children were all grown-up. They acted as though they knew that somehow I would figure out solutions to these communication problems. All their lives they had had a mother who liked words, who liked putting them together, who enjoyed giving her children assistance in anything involving the use of words. And I suspect it must have seemed strange, if not a little frightening, to know that their mother was having to have professional help in an area she liked best: words and their use.

But coming from a family where laughter is usual, we concentrated on the funny parts of aphasia. They never acted embarrassed. Rather the children made a game of my difficulties. They had me entertain them by practicing words I was having trouble getting out – *grocery* is still a blinger. They tried not to help me too often. They didn't get annoyed with me. And an often repeated remark was, "Oh, Mother, you're so funny."

From the many aphasics and their families we have met,

talked with and enjoyed since my stroke, we have learned that impatience is apt to be rampant. In those instances where the aphasic and mate are both home all the time a valid reason for impatience could be too much togetherness. I know that I need time to myself; so does Hans. But then our marriage has been geared to times apart from each other as he travels a good many weeks every year. Judging by those we've talked to, most aphasics want and need time to themselves just as their mates need time away from aphasia. Both of them should have it.

Often it isn't time alone each needs as much as time apart from each other. Time for recharging batteries that have been run down –time with friends or shopping or sitting watching people. Quiet time for listening to bird song and enjoying the beauties of flowers. We understand there are cities with facilities, sometimes just for stroke patients, where an aphasic can be brought to spend the day. In these places there are activities, meals, arrangements for resting, friends to talk to or just to sit with and enjoy. And this gives the mate a number of hours to attend to all kinds of things including a time for forgetting and relaxation. These times away from each other can be the ticket ensuring the ability to cope reasonably well. Even brief periods may be helpful – a walk, digging in the yard, a chat and a cup of coffee with a neighbor, soaking in the bathtub fortified with a tall drink and a good story. There are as many ways to get around this thorny problem as there are aphasics and their mates. Only sometimes it takes a lot of digging – a lot of help to find workable solutions.

The Quality of Help Accorded to Us by Professionals

To the professional people who took care of me go more plusses than minuses. There were two who felt I didn't fit a proper pattern. But then they may not have had enough experience with aphasics to know that there is no pattern. We are all different. No overall rules. Yes, indeed, we're quite a challenge. The only professional I really wanted was the speech therapist. Having her brought only joy and a good feeling that accomplishment was possible.

From some of the things we've heard in the past few years we know there are instances where families have been brushed aside as though they were unimportant, unintelligent, nothing but a nuisance. We hope those instances are rare. The family may need as much shoring up as the patient. They, also, need direction. They need information. They need as much layman's knowledge about aphasia as they are willing to absorb. They, too, need encouragement and loving touches and smiles.

My aphasia is 8 years old and coping continues. Why shouldn't it? Problem solving adds flavor to life, puts zing into a day, helps us achieve more internal growth than a quiet drifting which can easily turn subdued acceptance into boredom.

Coping means figuring what things I'm ready to try next. I'm not a devoted-to-the-kitchen female but lately I've experimented with rolls, lemon pie, and a special birthday cake. Results were o.k. and it felt good to know that after an absence of 8 years I still can bake these gastronomic delights. The accomplishment that pleased me most was being able to put on an apron and tie it behind my back. It took awhile but my right hand didn't fumble in space or make too many bobbles.

Life in toto flies along fairly smoothly. The children say they forget I'm an aphasic until they get a letter from me which hasn't been re-read and corrected. Then they realize anew. If I'm hurrying to type them all sorts of this's and thats I leave out syllables, I add syllables, I mention one idea, then mix it with another one until getting a letter from Mother means deciphering a strange code.

I find that coping with aphasia has some sterling attributes: a deeper appreciation of my husband; a delight in the sensitivity and perceptions of our children; good feelings when surrounded by the understanding and love of friends; fun meeting people with a few of the same difficulties; the joy of having new friends some of whom I know only through lively correspondence. And there has been an inner growth bringing me a serenity which comes from my feeling, my knowing that my brain may be finite, but my mind is gloriously infinite.

Why do I say my aphasia is forever? At this point many people I meet do not know I'm an aphasic. Heavens! They don't even know the word. Much less what it means. But, you see, one of the sneaky sides of aphasia is that there are difficulties only the aphasic may know – things which are not visible to anyone else but with which he must contend day in and day out. I will tell you about some of those gluey difficulties leading me to know that aphasia sticks to me like a shadow.

Making instant decisions is a problem. It never used to be.

It can lead to funny experiences. At home I handle the behind-the-scenes details for our business. And sometimes there are calls from manufacturers when Hans is on the road selling. These calls necessitate minor decisions and it is doubtful if any of the callers realize my predicament. One day I had three such calls in quick succession. When they were successfully completed I heaved a sigh of relief only to have the phone ring again. This was a persistent telephone seller and I heard myself say, "I can't say no and I can't say yes. I can't decide. I'm an aphasic." From the caller came a startled "Oh" and quickly she hung up. All by myself I had a wonderful laugh.

I am still pretty much tied to doing one thing at a time. The other day I was attempting to wrap a package which I can do with a great deal of concentration. While doing this I was asked a question. And I found myself just standing, not only not wrapping the package or answering the question, but really not thinking about either one. Not thinking about anything. Or say I'm attending a tea where I'm expected to mingle with guests and converse. I'd better not have anything to eat or drink or my interacting will be nil.

There is a huge empty space I fall into when too many stimuli have impinged on me at once. Then for a moment I'm a blank, an unhappy blank, as I wonder what in the world is going on and how do I get out of this unpleasant, nothing place. I seem to need a structured life. Several weeks ago our sons were coming for dinner. I had made plans for where we would eat. I hadn't counted on one of them bringing a friend. Which was fine. Only the plans I had made were not workable. And the food was at the every-thing-ready-at-once stage. I couldn't think. I didn't know where a table cloth was. I simply didn't know what was happening or what I should do about it. It was a bad blank spot. Hans stepped in and got everything going the proper way. Not many years ago, during market weeks, there were times when I would work all day, come home and have as many as 25 or 30 people for dinner. And I enjoyed it! Today, one tiny change can leave me temporarily *non compos mentis*.

There is an invisible cord around my throat making talking feel like I am having to push against tight rubber bands in order for words to emerge. I have to tell myself what it is I want to say and sometimes, if I'm weary, the combination of having to direct my thinker and having to work to get things spoken results in a bunch of blah. Or nothing.

Misinterpreting what has been said to me probably bothers me the most. The funniest example was when I thought a doctor had told me that I had an extra room in my head. The errors I catch today aren't as glaring or amusing as that, but I have to be careful about repeating things I've heard because sometimes remembered conversations are peculiar enough for me to know they aren't coming back to me as they really were.

It is disconcerting to suddenly be unable to remember how to do a simple thing like getting out of the bathtub or how to make gravy. Instead of poking the panic button, I relax in the tub until the solution pops in my head. Or I do some other task until the formula for making gravy comes out of hiding.

If I'm listening to a talk or reading something interesting what I'm apt to remember is the last sentence I heard or the last sentence I read. And probably not too long at that. I may not be able to hear the talk again but I can always re-read the book, and it is true that while these things were happening I was enjoying. Which is more important to me than how much of it I retain.

I have to consciously give instructions to my right arm and leg. The leg *will* drag if not told what to do – what to avoid, what to step over, when to step up or down. The arm acts like an extra appendage stuck on me any old which way and does nothing. I constantly need to remember to tell my arm to do things. It's fairly good about doing what it's told but it almost never does anything voluntarily. It has to be reminded.

There are seconds which seem like hours when my swallower won't work. Or unwanted times when swallowing induces choking. But amusing note: I can't gargle. By the time I have instructed muscles either I'm sputtering or the gargling stuff has gone down. Functions once deemed automatic from the throat on down, literally from top to bottom, no longer can be always depended on. Sometimes those processes of intake and outgo have to have specific instructions. And sometimes I have no proper control. Unpleasant effects of stroke which have to be contended with as gracefully as possible.

These tell you some of the quirks of my aphasia. Something very different may be another aphasic's nemesis. Ideas I think about roll along in my head at a good clip. The words I say aloud have to be sent through a not always reliable computer and pushed out. Need one wonder why fatigue besets many aphasics? The cerebral acrobatics we must employ to present a reasonable semblance of "normality" is far greater than most suspect.

It is awesome to realize what onslaughts to the body and the brain man can survive. And awesome to watch the will he demonstrates as he copes. Many an aphasic displays an effective combination of will and optimism tied with a beautiful sense of humor. Which doesn't mean he expects miracles. For, deep in his heart, the aphasic usually knows how permanent is his aphasia.

He also must be aware of the helpful factors which are a part of his continual relearning: self-discipline which means a daily regimen of speech and physical therapy ensuring him a viable life; acceptance of his aphasia by the use of the many abilities left to him despite being stroked; and an awareness of the moment to moment beauty in nature and people. These ensure him comfort in his family and his circle of friends, and provide him with real growth. And that kind of growth never needs to stop.

Helen Harlan Wulf was born in Chicago, and attended Northwestern University, where she was elected to Phi Beta Kappa and received a B.A. degree in 1935. She holds the M.A. degree in Sociology (1958) from Southern Methodist University.

Mrs. Wulf now lives in Dallas, Texas, where she has for more than twenty years been associated with her husband in his business as a manufacturers' sales representative in children's apparel.

The book was designed by Donald R. Ross. The typeface for the text is Times Roman, the design of which was supervised by Stanley Morison; and the display face is Ultra Bodoni.

The text is printed on Natural text paper and the book is bound in Permalin Book Covering cloth over binder's boards. Manufactured in the United States of America.